MW01488908

A SQUIRRELLY ADVENTURE

AMANDA JEAN

Book Design: **Amanda Jean** and **Israel Lopez**

Editor: **Kimberlie Neathery**

Illustrations: **Lori Block**

2018: Second Edition

Copyright © 2018 Amanda Jean.

All rights reserved. No part of this book may be used or reproduced by any means, graphic, electronic, or mechanical, including photocopying, recording, taping or by any information storage retrieval system without the written permission of the author except in the case of brief quotations embodied in critical articles and reviews.

Balboa Press books may be ordered through booksellers or by contacting:

Balboa Press
A Division of Hay House
1663 Liberty Drive
Bloomington, IN 47403
www.balboapress.com
1 (877) 407-4847

Because of the dynamic nature of the Internet, any web addresses or links contained in this book may have changed since publication and may no longer be valid. The views expressed in this work are solely those of the author and do not necessarily reflect the views of the publisher, and the publisher hereby disclaims any responsibility for them.

Any people depicted in stock imagery provided by Getty Images are models, and such images are being used for illustrative purposes only.
Certain stock imagery © Getty Images.

ISBN: 978-1-9822-0695-6 (sc)
978-1-9822-0696-3 (e)

Library of Congress Control Number: 2018907258

Print information available on the last page.

Balboa Press rev. date: 07/16/2018

BALBOA
PRESS
A DIVISION OF HAY HOUSE

To my heavenly Father
and to all of my family and friends for your continued support
and love for me, even though I'm a lil' nutty.

"When you're curious, you find lots of interesting things to do."
- Walt Disney

NUTTY NOTES

EXPLORE!
BE NUTTY AND HAVE FUN!

A SQUIRRELLY ADVENTURE

Written by:
Amanda Jean

Illustrated by:
Lori Block

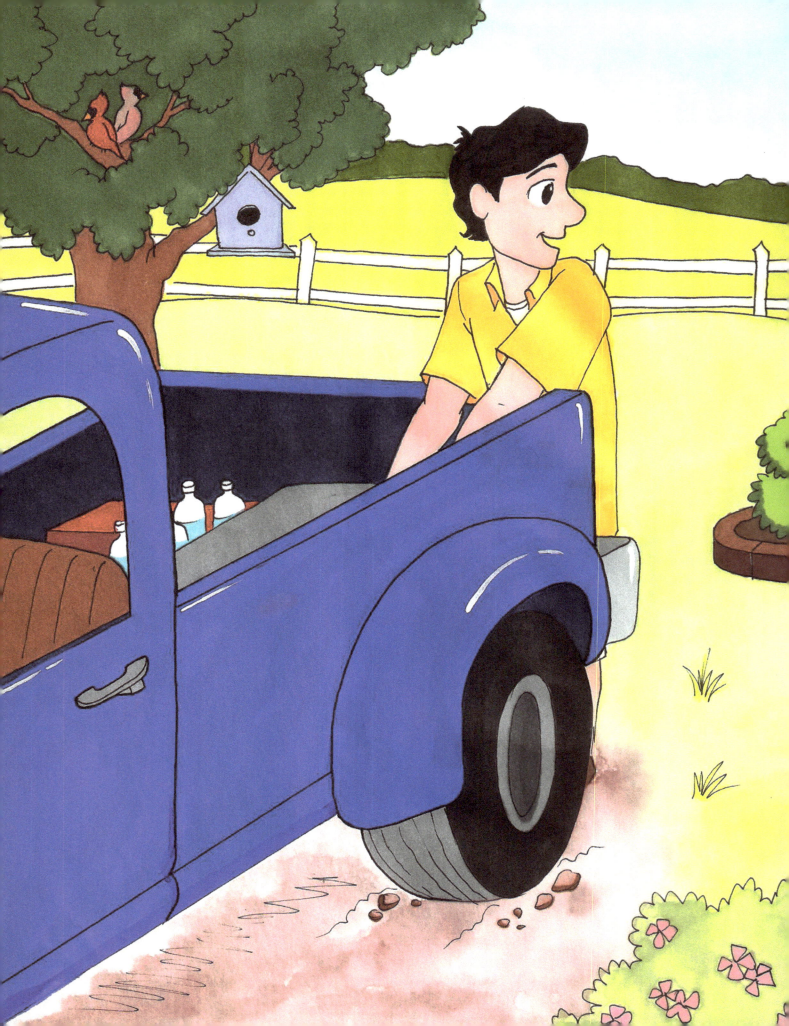

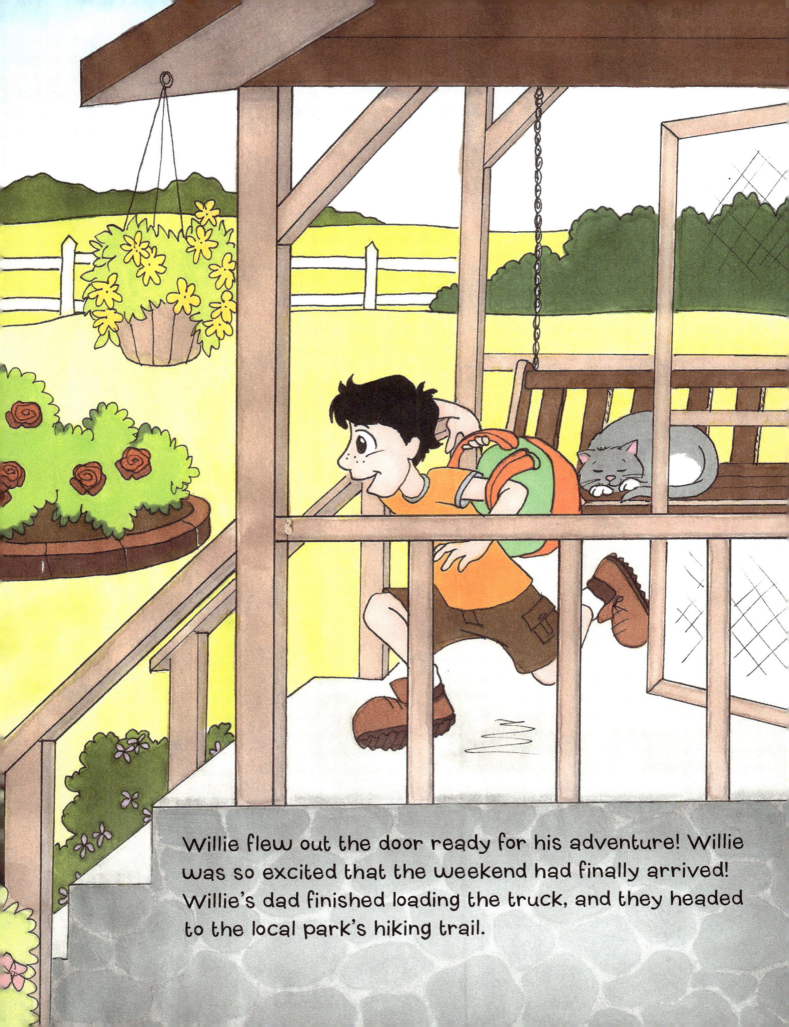

Willie flew out the door ready for his adventure! Willie was so excited that the weekend had finally arrived! Willie's dad finished loading the truck, and they headed to the local park's hiking trail.

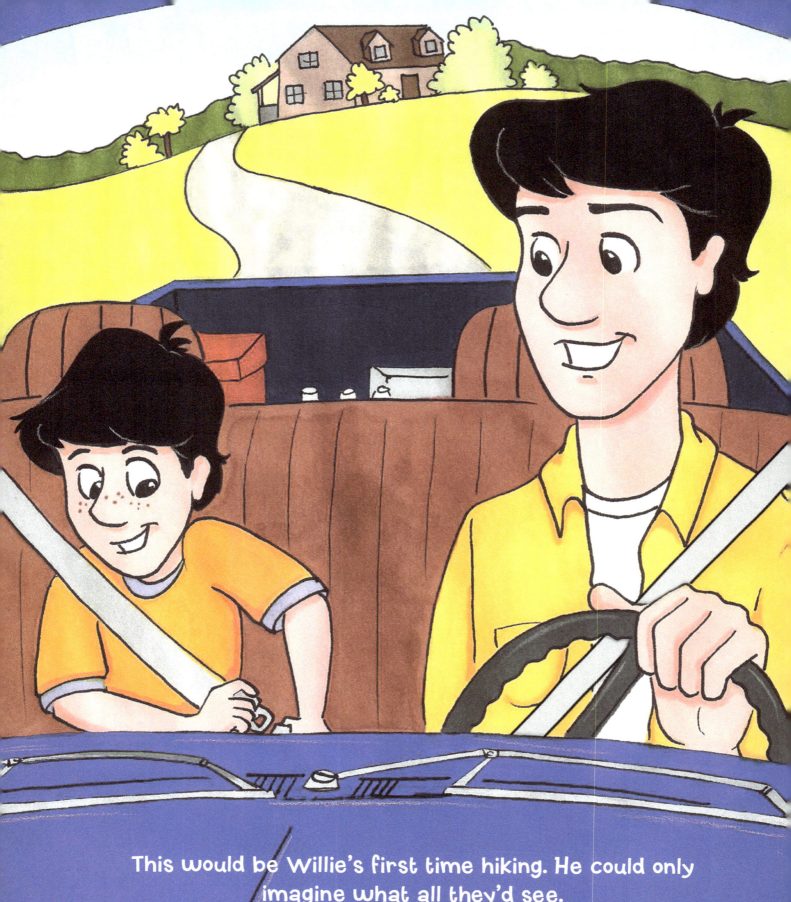

This would be Willie's first time hiking. He could only imagine what all they'd see.

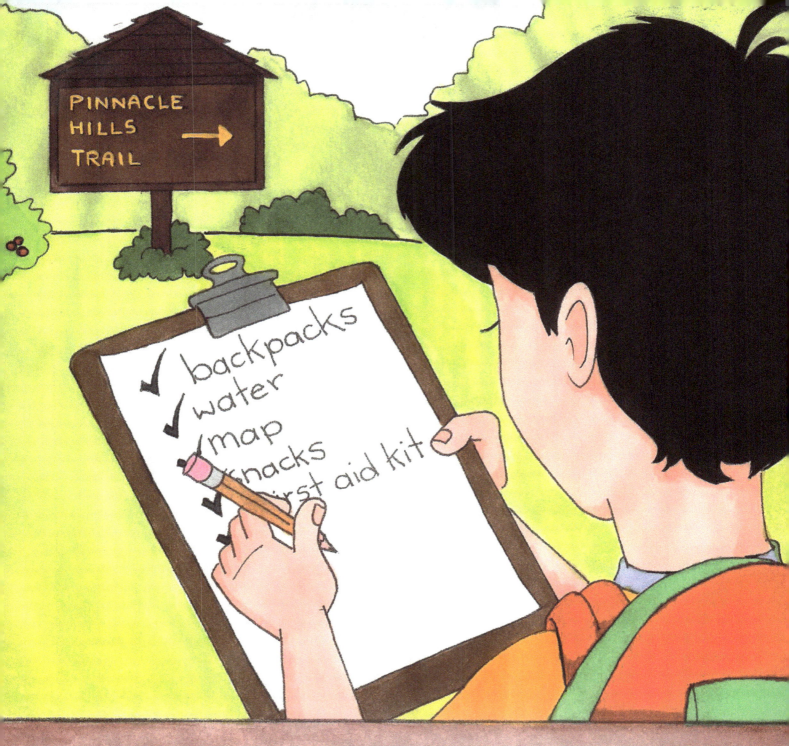

They finally arrived!

Willie sat on a bench near the entrance to the trail and studied his list.

Backpack √
Water √
Map √
Snacks √
First-aid kit √

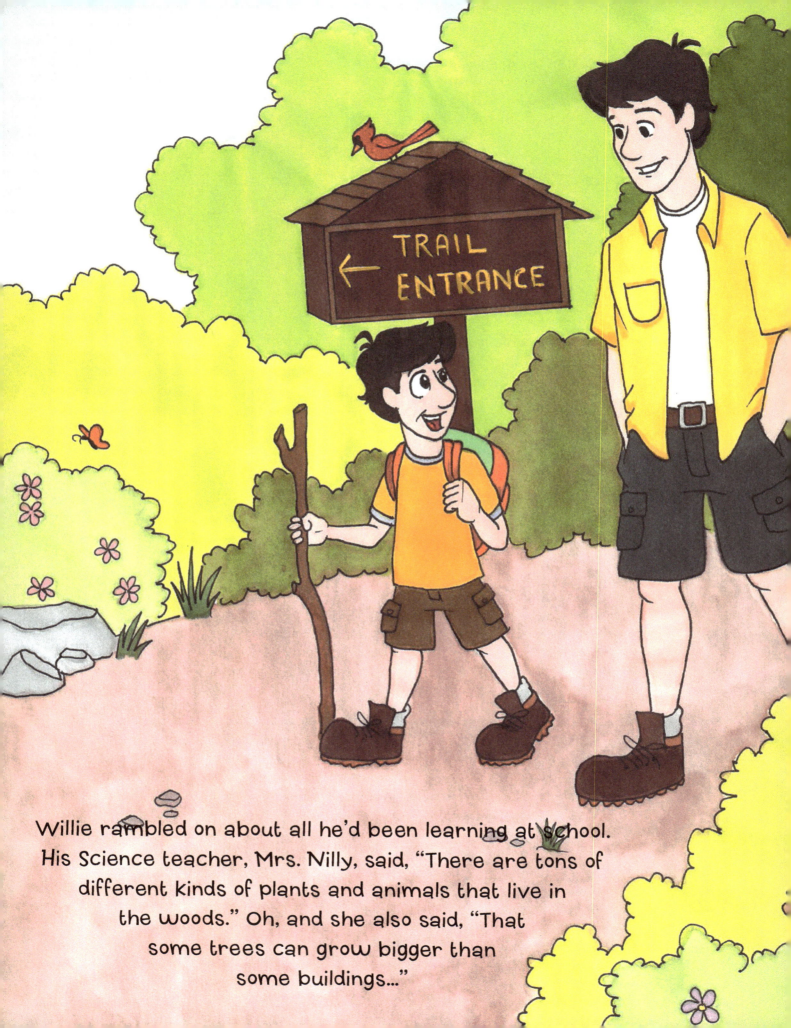

Willie rambled on about all he'd been learning at school. His Science teacher, Mrs. Nilly, said, "There are tons of different kinds of plants and animals that live in the woods." Oh, and she also said, "That some trees can grow bigger than some buildings…"

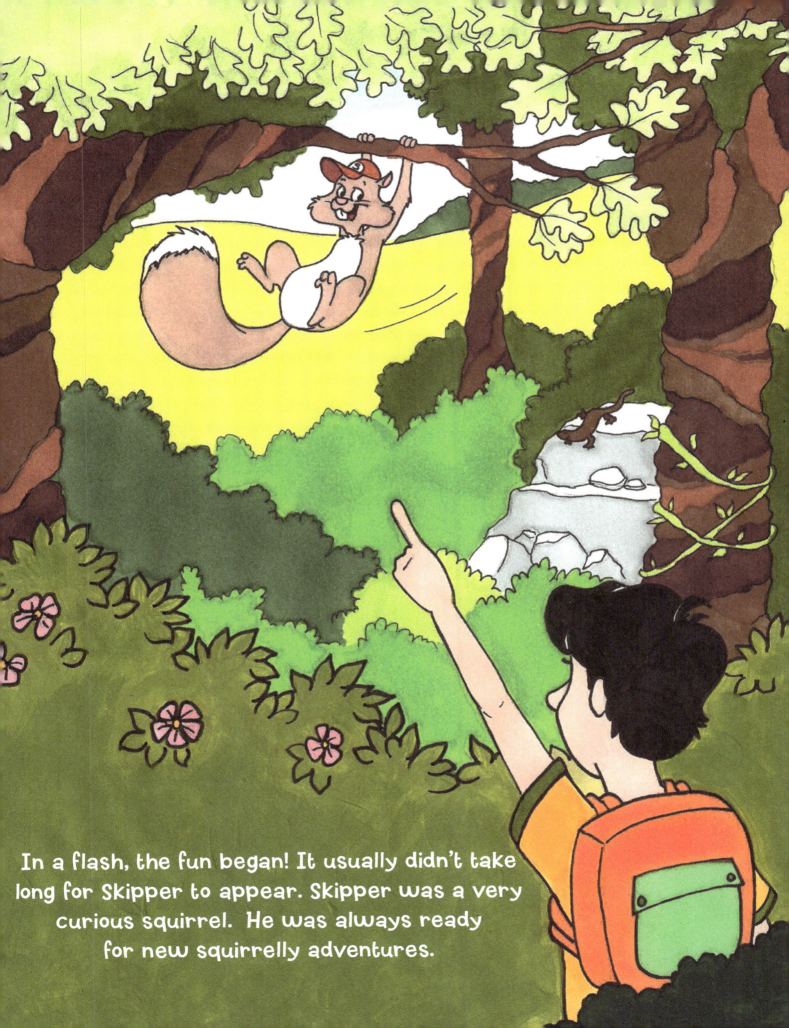

In a flash, the fun began! It usually didn't take long for Skipper to appear. Skipper was a very curious squirrel. He was always ready for new squirrelly adventures.

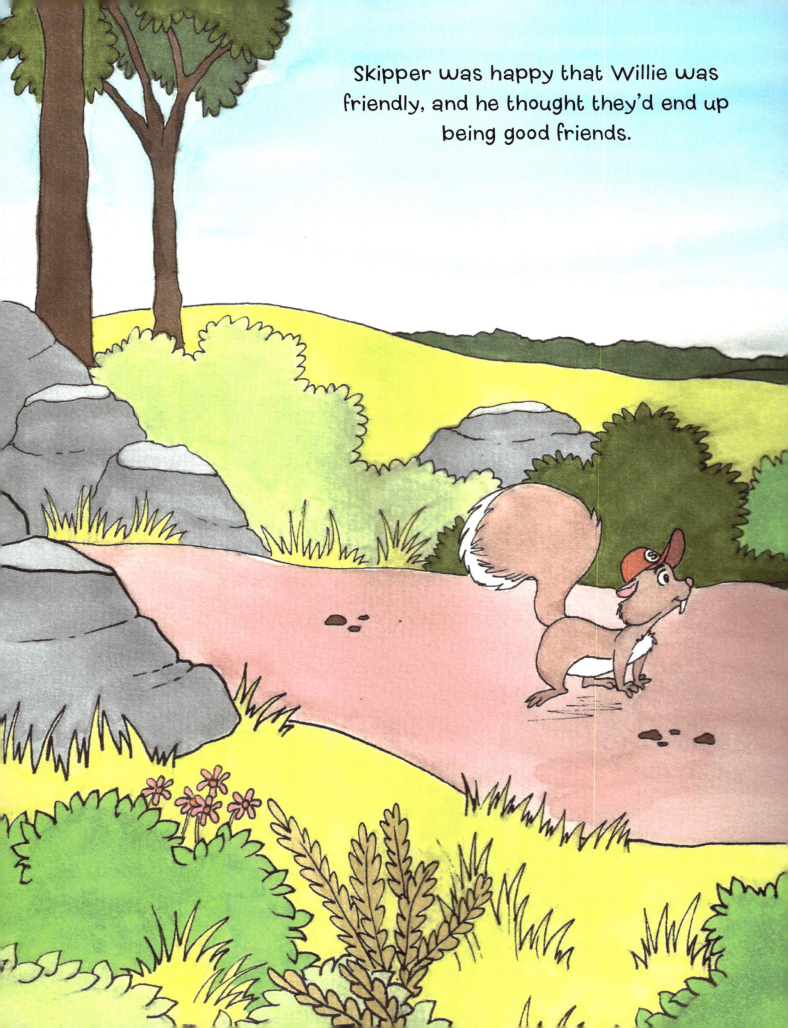

Skipper was happy that Willie was friendly, and he thought they'd end up being good friends.

Skipper saw B.J. the bluejay coming to make his presence known. B.J. squawked and squawked but Skipper didn't notice him because he was busy with his new friend, Willie.

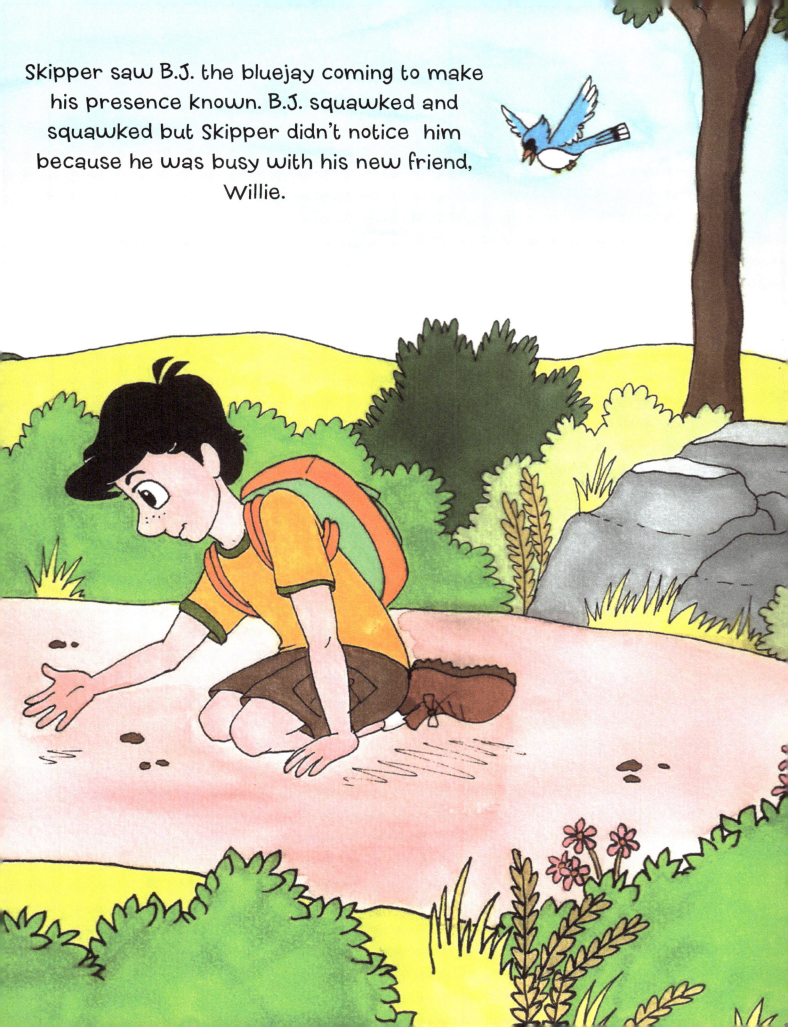

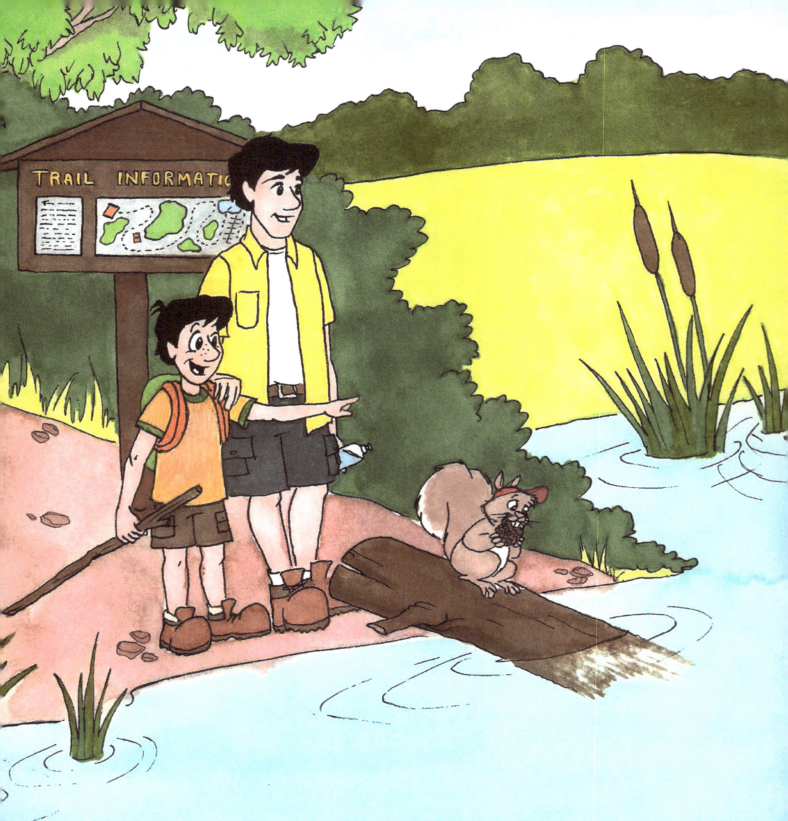

The trail led them to a small pond. Skipper hopped onto a log for a quick snack. All of a sudden they heard a loud splash and saw a huge fish jumping from the water.

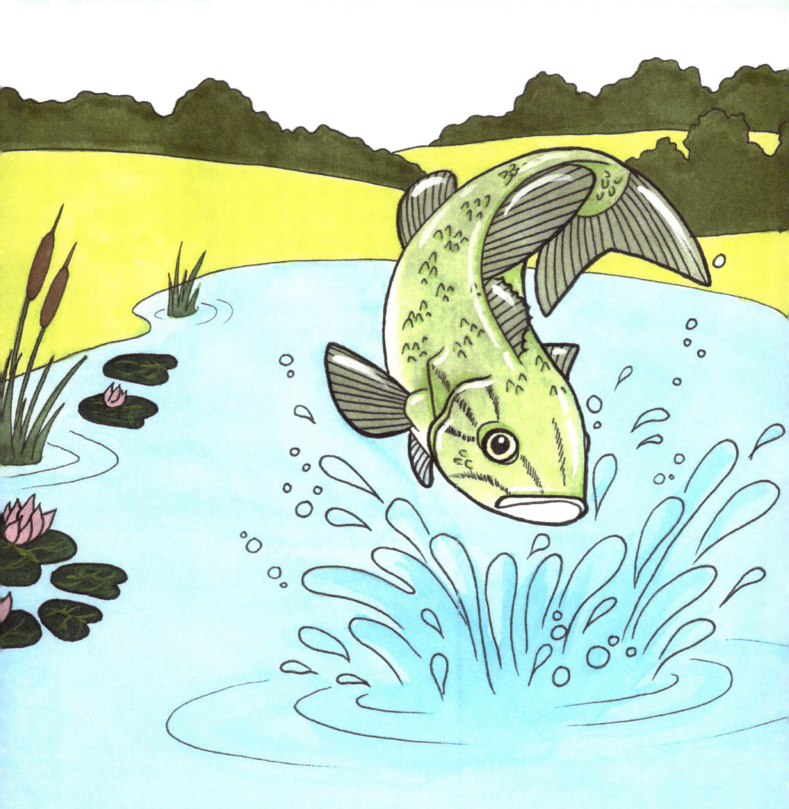

Willie's school teacher had recently taught his class about different kinds of fish. Willie proudly told his dad, "That to know what kind of fish it is, you need to know what type of water he lives in, then you count his fins, and then you look at the color of his skin. Yep! It's a largemouth bass!"

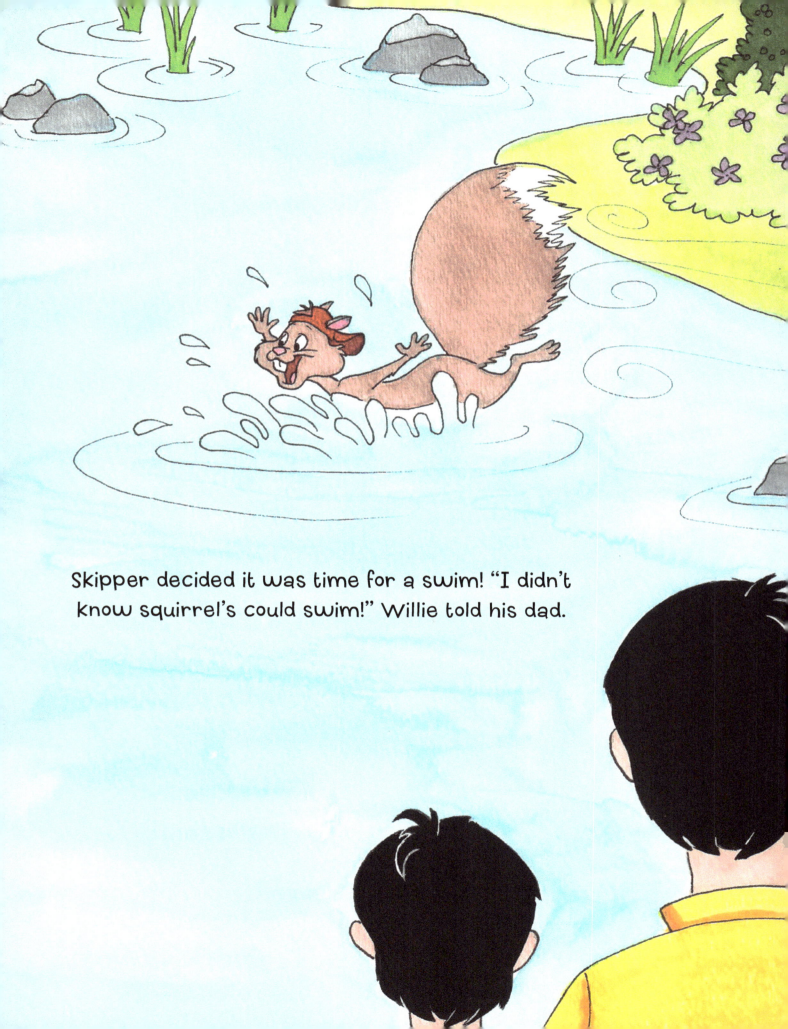

Skipper decided it was time for a swim! "I didn't know squirrel's could swim!" Willie told his dad.

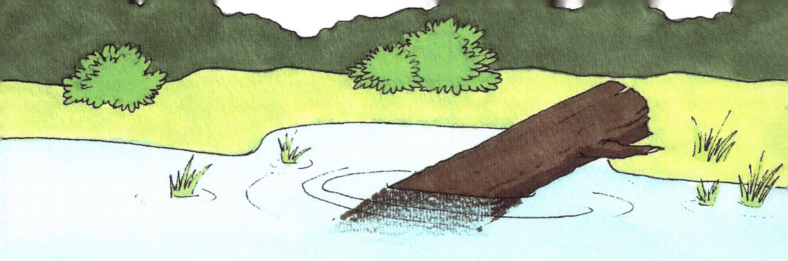

A friendly frog had lost his way while searching for something to eat. Skipper said, "Hop on, and I'll give you a ride across the creek."

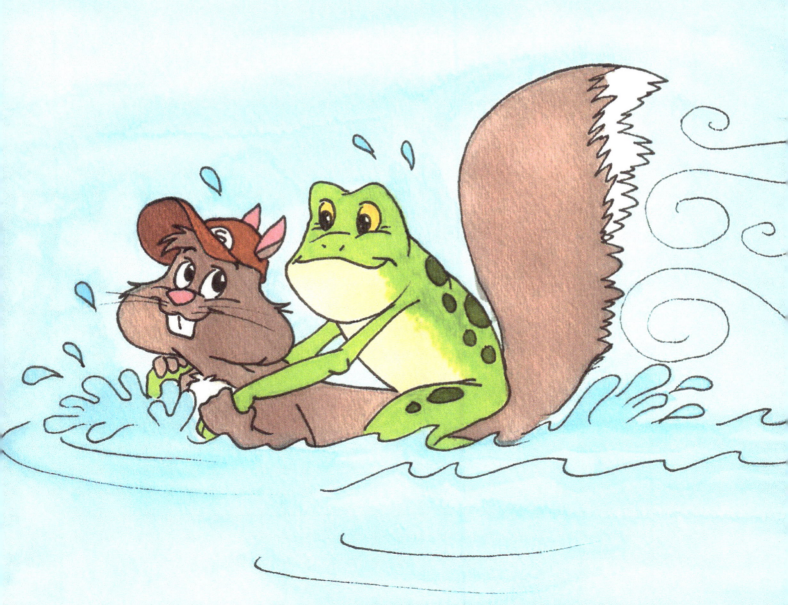

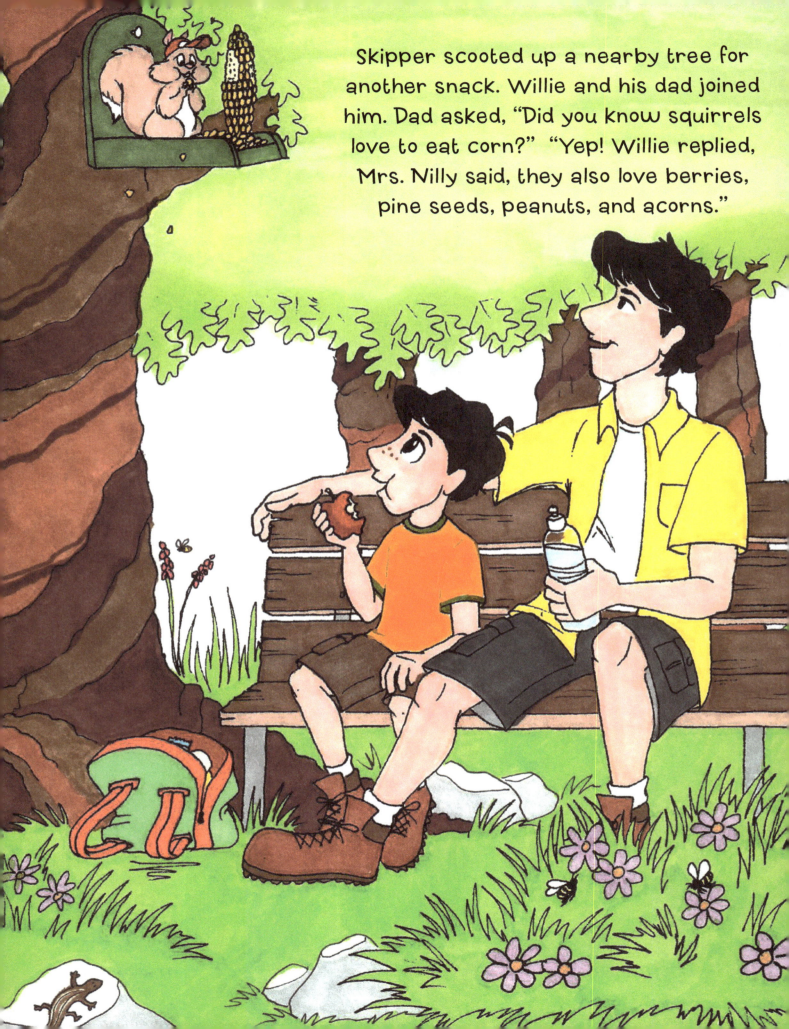

Skipper scooted up a nearby tree for another snack. Willie and his dad joined him. Dad asked, "Did you know squirrels love to eat corn?" "Yep! Willie replied, Mrs. Nilly said, they also love berries, pine seeds, peanuts, and acorns."

A man and his dog were enjoying the trail. The man stopped and told Willie and his dad about a really cool waterfall up ahead. The man said, "I'd be careful though, it's slick". Willie thanked the man, and promised to be careful, and took off in search of the waterfall.

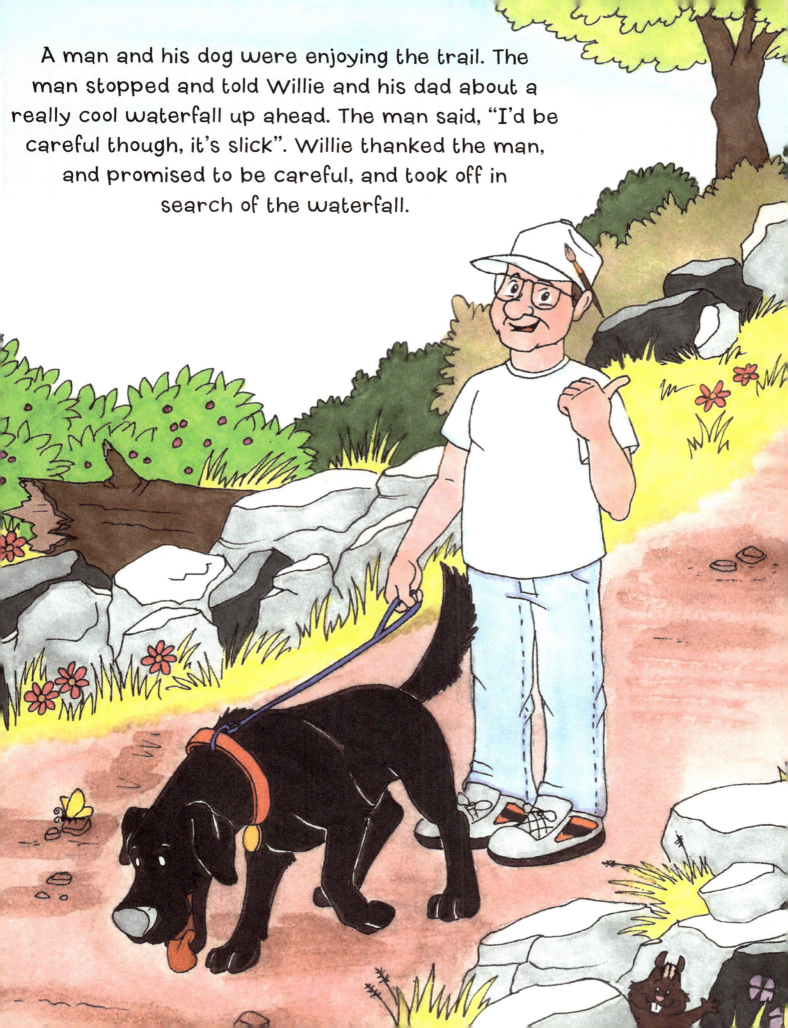

Skipper hopped onto Willie's lap to hear all about the cool waterfall they'd see.

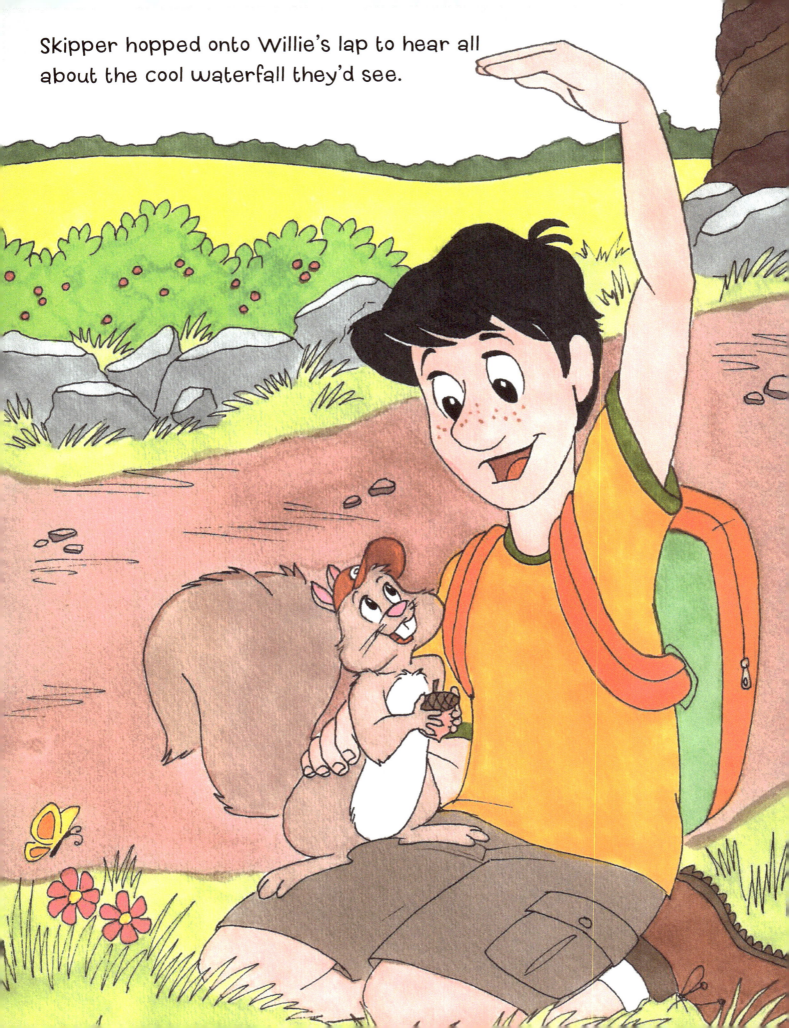

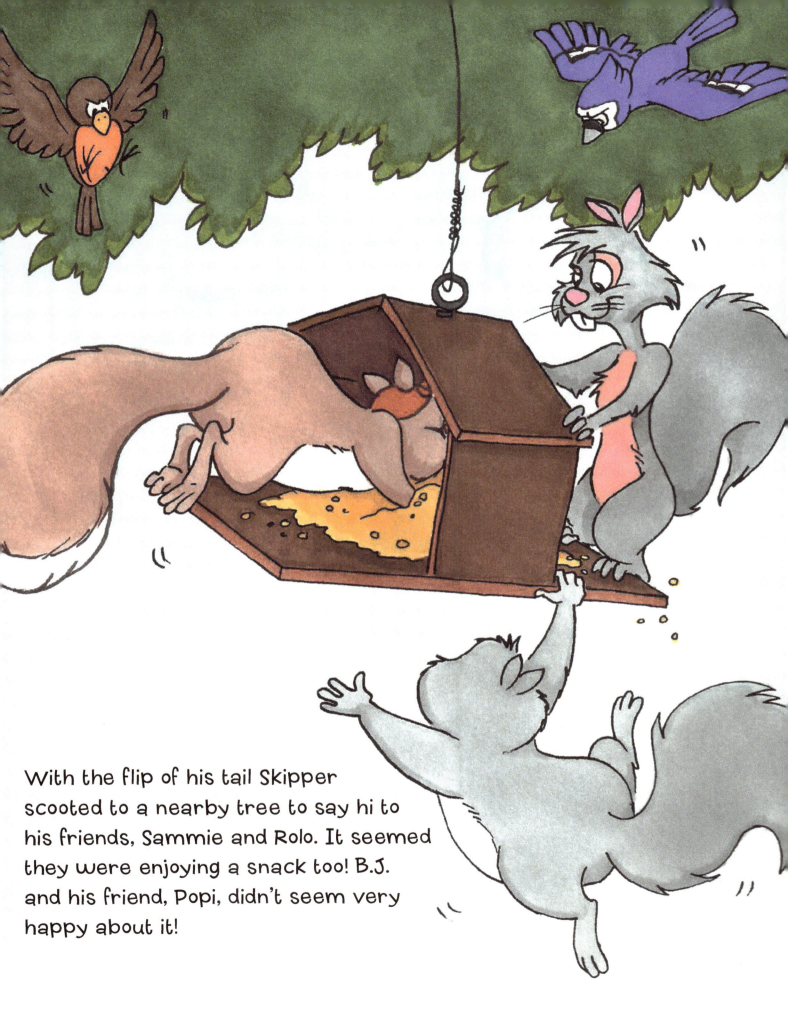

With the flip of his tail Skipper scooted to a nearby tree to say hi to his friends, Sammie and Rolo. It seemed they were enjoying a snack too! B.J. and his friend, Popi, didn't seem very happy about it!

Once their bellies were full, they hung out in their favorite tree. Skipper made sure to say "hi" to his friend, Billie Jean. Skipper didn't hang out long, he didn't want to miss going with Willie to see the waterfall.

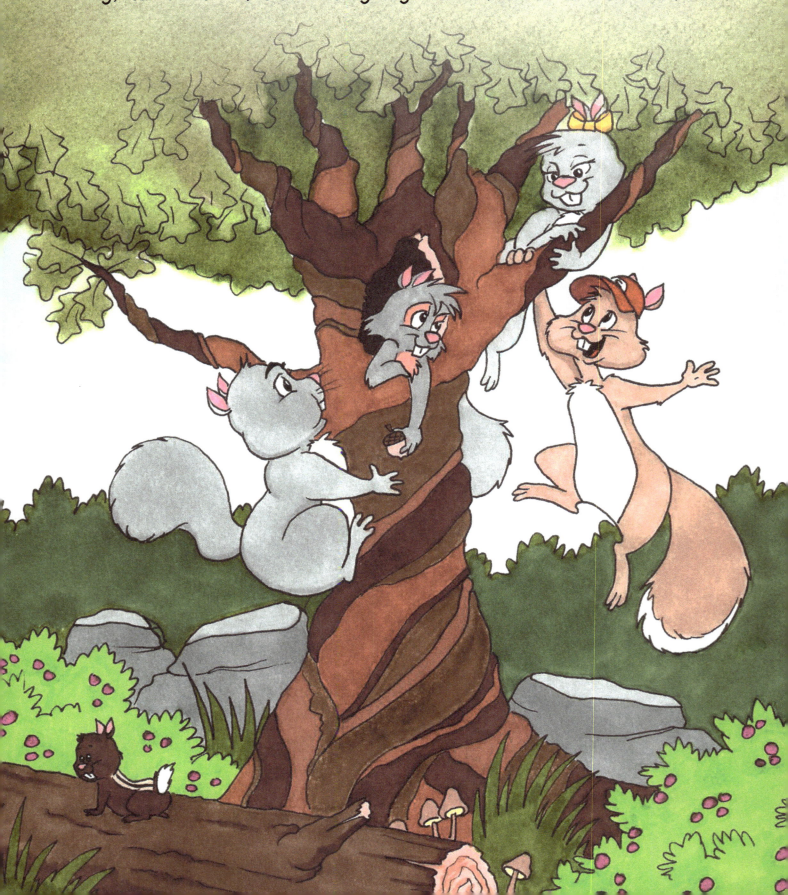

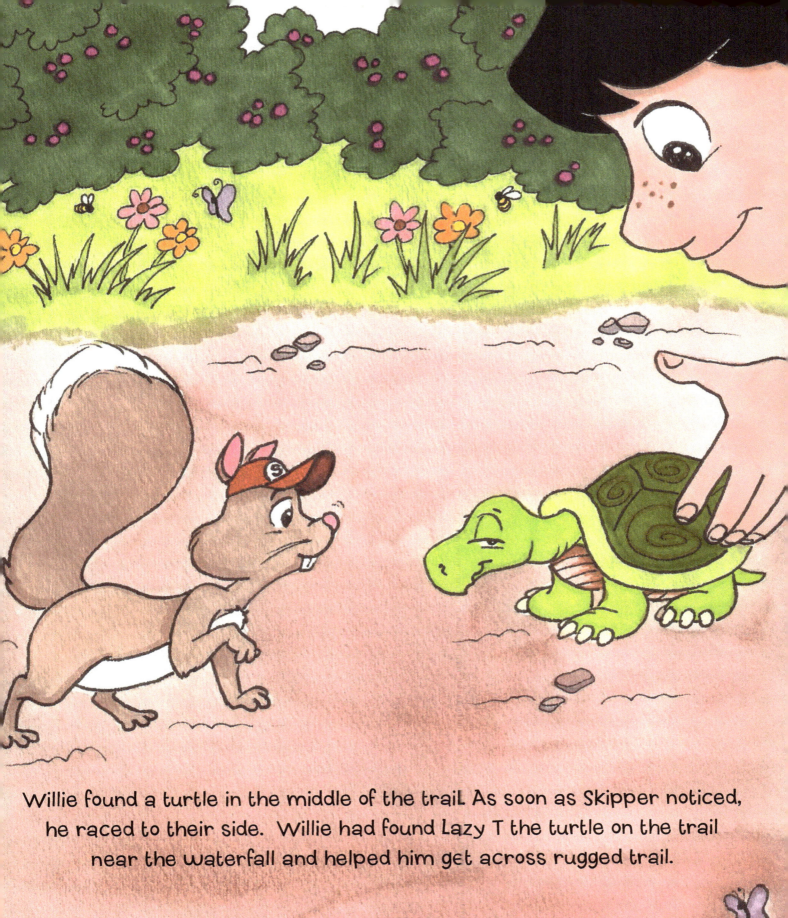

Willie found a turtle in the middle of the trail As soon as Skipper noticed, he raced to their side. Willie had found Lazy T the turtle on the trail near the waterfall and helped him get across rugged trail.

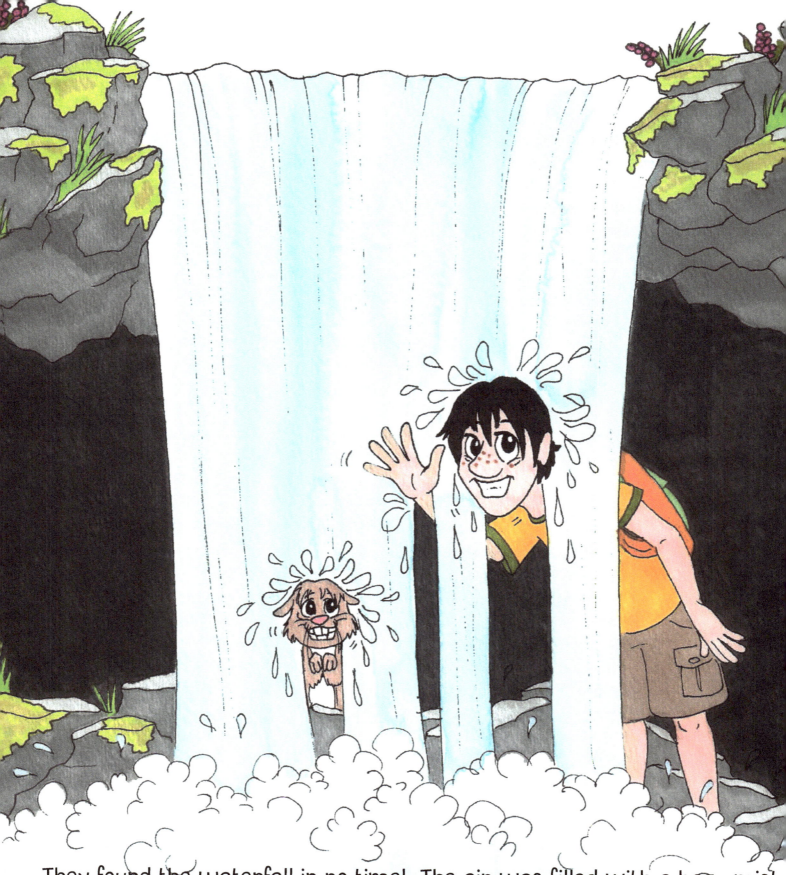

They found the waterfall in no time! The air was filled with a hazy mist
and the water was very cold. They explored a narrow path that led
to a cave. Inside the cave, the walls and rocks were covered
with green algae that looked like gooey slime.

Willie and Skipper shook off the cold mountain water
and headed back to the trail.

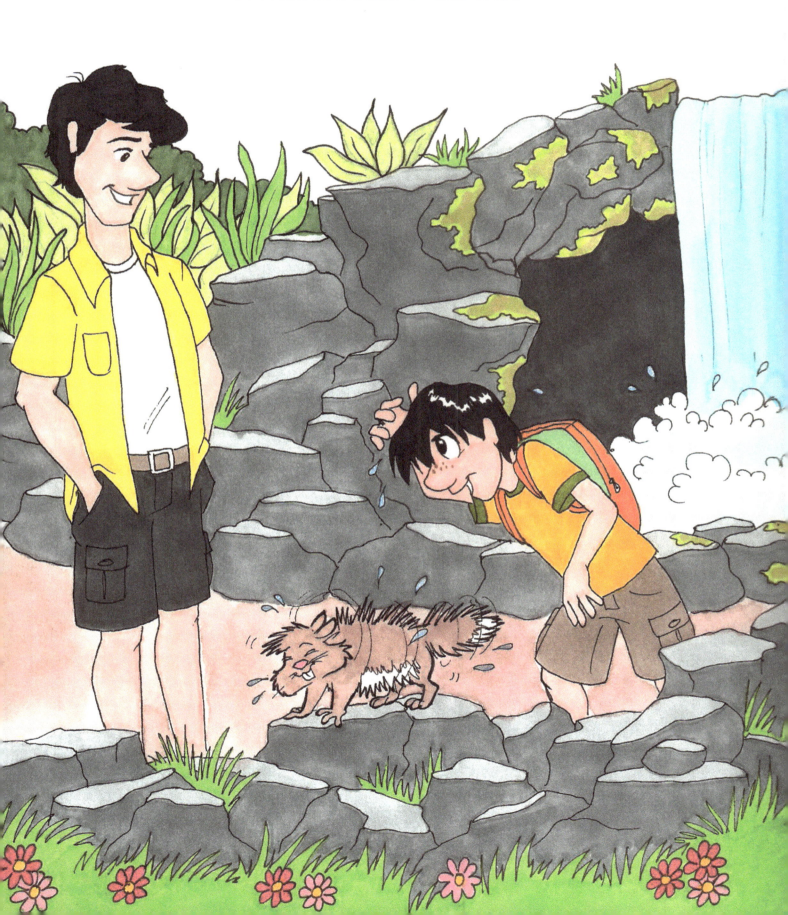

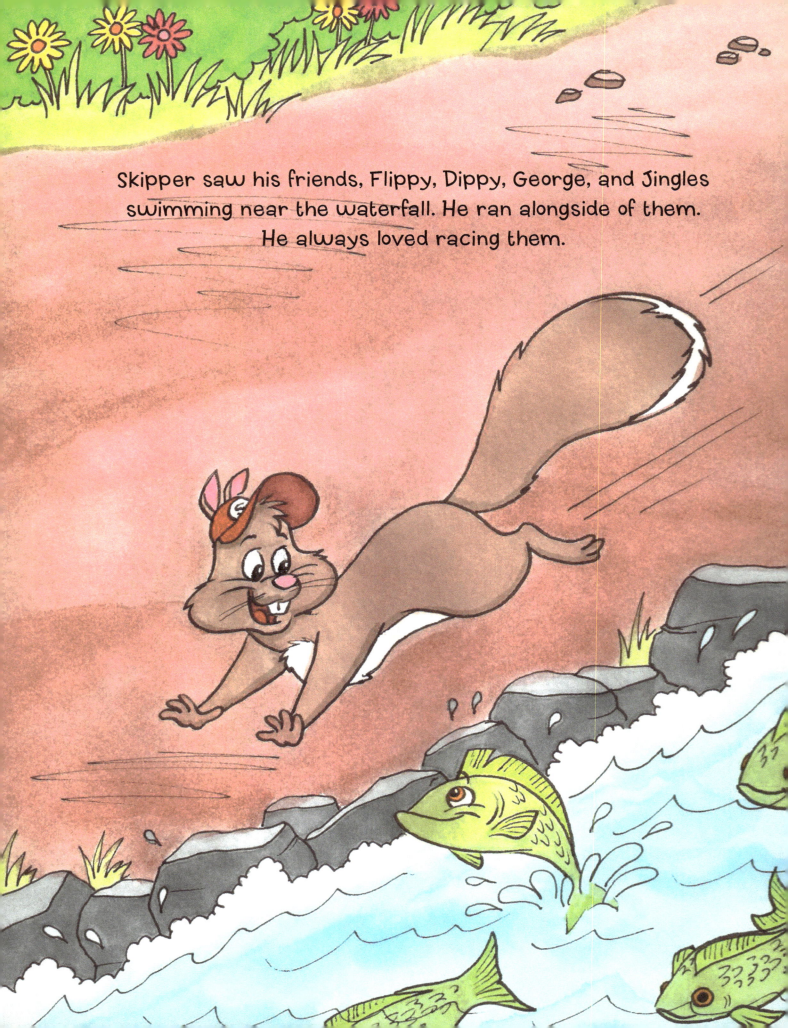

Skipper saw his friends, Flippy, Dippy, George, and Jingles swimming near the waterfall. He ran alongside of them. He always loved racing them.

Willie and his dad stopped to pick a couple of flowers to take home to Willie's mother. She always loved getting flowers.

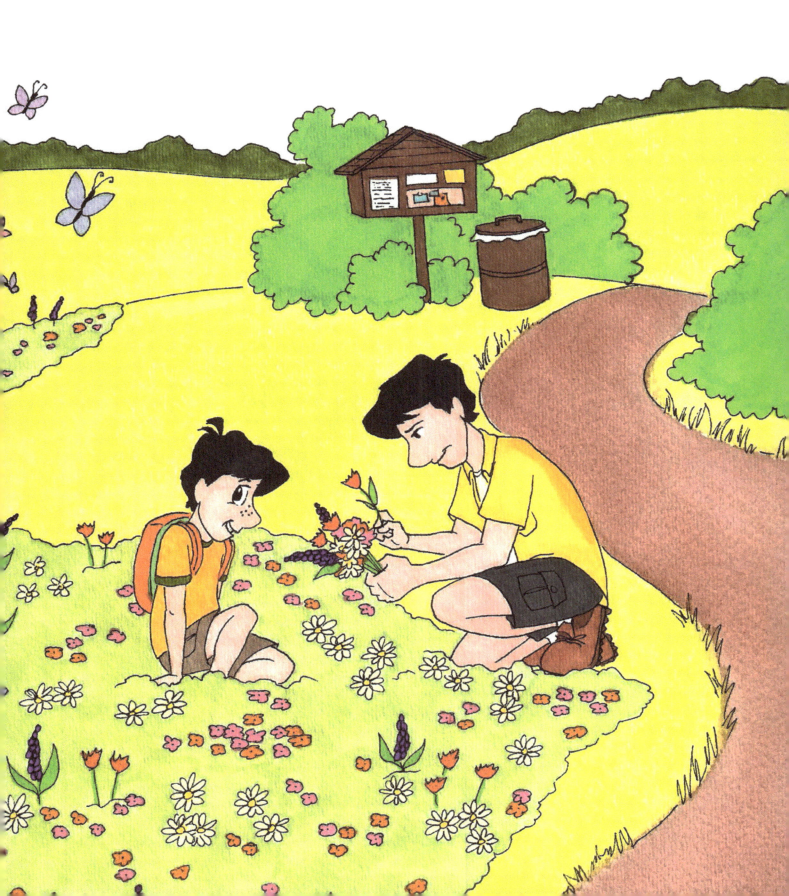

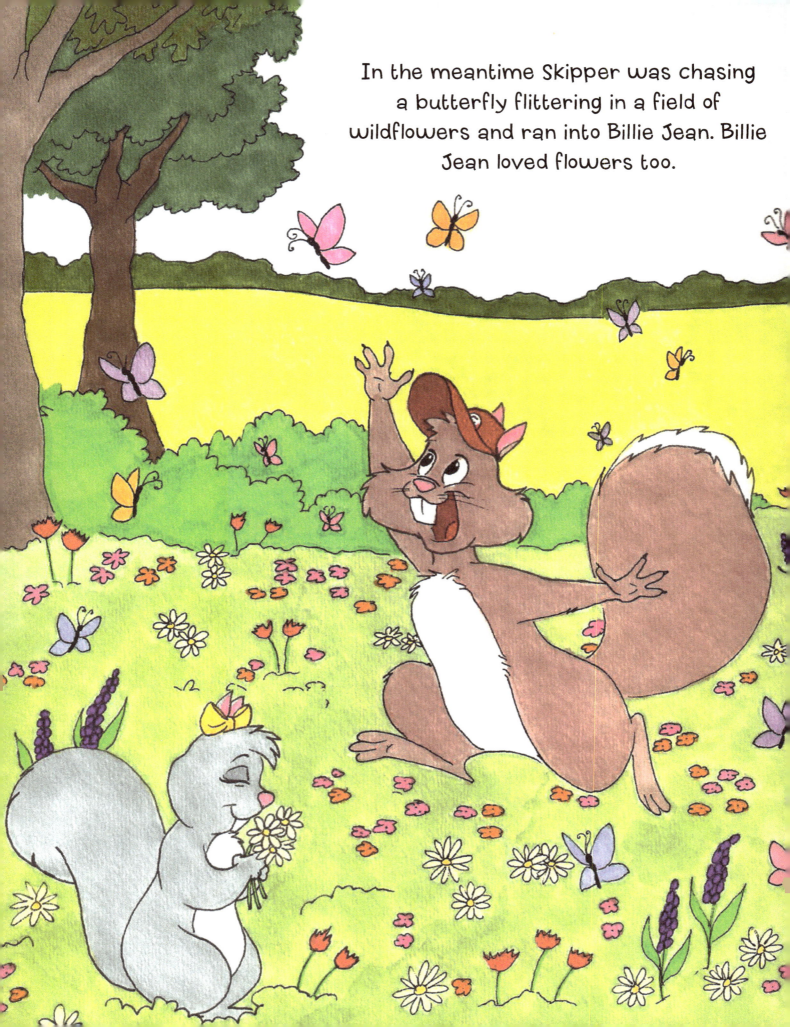

In the meantime Skipper was chasing a butterfly flittering in a field of wildflowers and ran into Billie Jean. Billie Jean loved flowers too.

The trail had come to an end. Willie and Skipper were now fast friends.

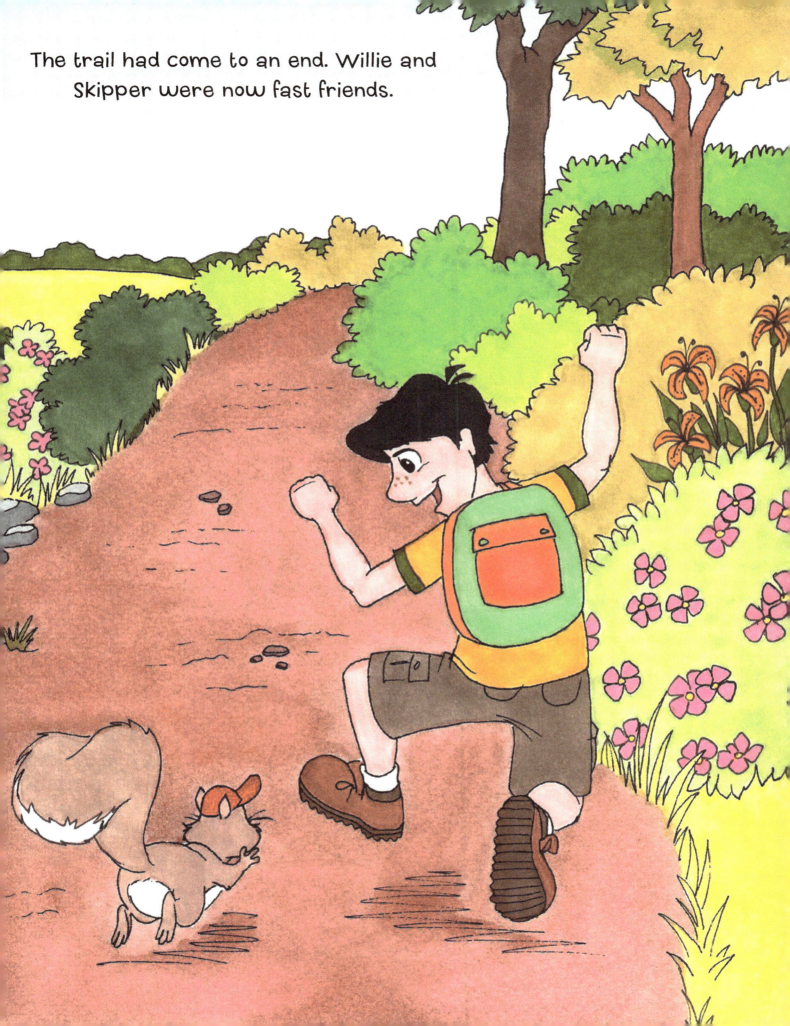

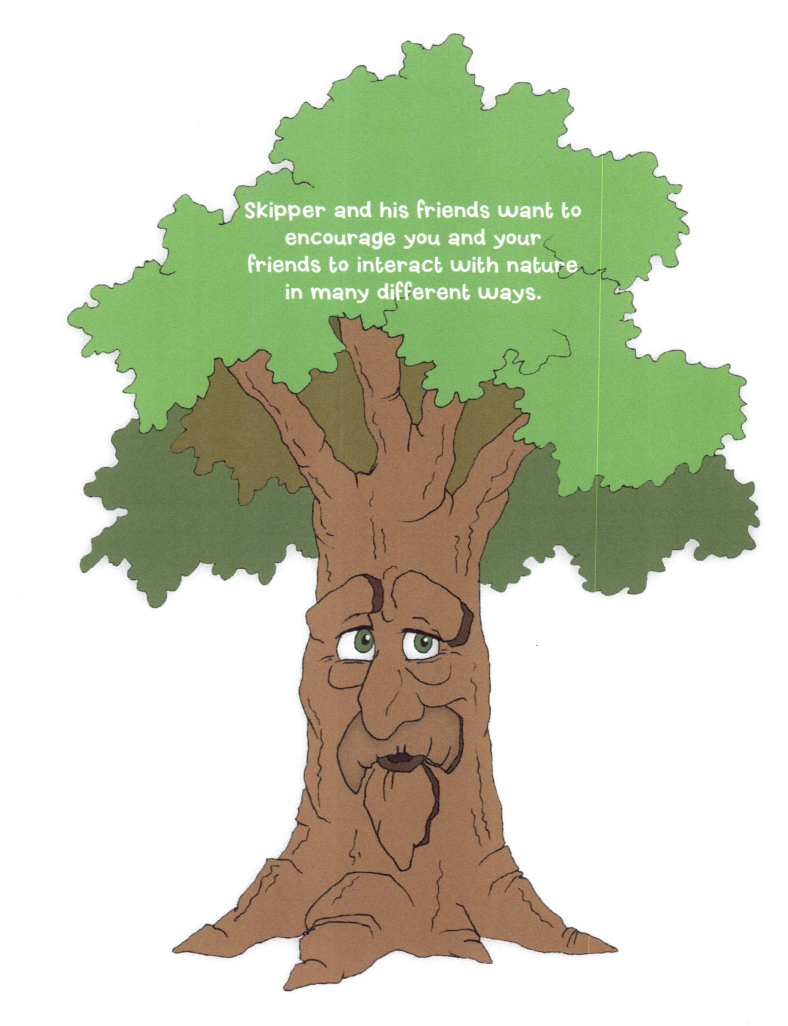

ABOUT THE AUTHOR

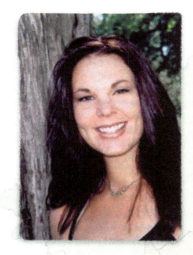

Amanda Jean has always had a spot in her heart for expressing her emotions through writing. Amanda created Skipper the Squirrel shortly after the birth of her first daughter. During this time she lived in scenic Northwest Arkansas, which provided her with the inspiration to write the book. In 2011, Amanda graduated from the University of Arkansas at Little Rock majoring in professional and technical writing and media production and design. She currently resides in Central Arkansas with her husband and their three daughters. She is in the process of developing an animated television series and companion website built around the character of Skipper the Squirrel.

ABOUT THE ILLUSTRATOR

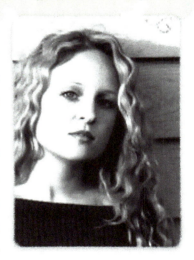

Lori Block began illustrating children's books at the age of 14, when a noted author visited her school and saw some of her artworks. She was hired on the spot for his next project and has since completed five children's books, all of which can be found in bookstores nationwide. A native of Waldenburg, Arkansas, Ms. Block received her bachelor of fine art from Arkansas State University in 2002. She resides in Jonesboro, Arkansas, and makes her living as a freelance artist. Aside from artwork, she enjoys many different interests and hobbies including traveling, playing the piano, reading, sewing, gardening, and even occasionally working on major movie sets. The setting and characters in Skipper appealed to her because of the many hours she has spent observing Arkansas wildlife while camping, hiking, and sitting on a tree stand in the "deer woods."

CPSIA information can be obtained
at www.ICGtesting.com
Printed in the USA
BVHW052109031118
532008BV00003B/3/P

Welcome to the family!

Creating a cookbook has been a lifetime in the making. While I'm only 32, that is still enough time to discover the joy and stress relief found in making something from "nothing." I do not claim to be a professional chef by any standard and have had no formal training in cooking. Everything is self-taught or earned through baking with the women (and a few men) in my family. The single most important thing learned from all those who instilled the passion for cooking is that whatever you're cooking must come from a place of love. Your heart must go into what you make or it will never have that "like grandma used to make" taste. With that in mind, this is a cookbook for everyday cooks feeding everyday people. This collection is geared towards appealing to most people's appetites. However, there are no gluten free, vegan, etc. recipes.

Many of these recipes are family recipes passed down at least 3 generations while others are of my own design and tweaking. You will see a few recipes in here that do not have exact measurements listed. This is because these recipes are only in my or the original cook's head. Welcome to the joy of cooking. Seasoning food is very subjective and half the fun is playing with spices to see what results. A helpful tip is to taste test as you go and add slowly and a little at a time until you are familiar with it. Cooking is truly an art so do not expect every recipe to turn out perfect the first time. Even the best cooks do not always get it right.

To help you pick out some of the "best" recipes included you will see a few recipes marked with a bee icon. These are the recipes that are favorites and/or frequently requested recipes.

I hope you enjoy these recipes as much as my family and friends have. May they warm your soul as much as they do your stomach.

Brandyn Rathman

1

Index

Introduction   1

Appetizers and Sides   3

Entrees   5

Crockpot Recipes   26

Baked Goods   33

Miscellaneous   48

Appetizers and Sides

- Little weenies
- Bacon weenies
- Cheesy pigs in a blanket
- Smoked mac n' cheese
- Grape salad
- Homemade egg noodles
- 7-layer dip
- Cinnamon apples
- Chicken Caesar pasta salad
- Fried okra
- Grilled cheese pull aparts
- Queso dip
- Italian rolls
- Baking powder biscuits
- Naan
- Cornbread
- Grandma D's olive dip
- Rose's crispy potatoes

LITTLE WEENIES

Ingredients	
1 jar grape jelly	1 package lil' weenies
1 jar chili sauce	

- Throw everything together in the crock pot and stir well (sounds odd but really does taste like BBQ sauce)
- Cook until thoroughly cooked
-

BACON WEENIES

Ingredients	
1 package bacon of your choice	Brown sugar
1 pack of lil' weenies	

- Preheat oven to 425 F
- Cut bacon into half or thirds (depending on how much bacon you want)
- Wrap bacon slice around weenie and use toothpick to keep in place
- Set wrapped weenies on baking sheet with parchment paper
- Sprinkle brown sugar on all weenies to coat thoroughly
- Cook until bacon to desired crispness, typically 15 minutes or so.

CHEESY PIGS IN A BLANKET

Ingredients	
1 pack. Crescent rolls	Melted butter
1 pack cheese filled lil' weenies	

- Preheat oven to temp indicated on crescent roll package
- Wrap lil' weenies in crescent roll dough and place on baking sheet
- Brush melted butter on all those piggies
- Cook for time specified on package of crescent rolls or until desired browning of dough

GRAPE SALAD

Ingredients	
Mix of red and green grapes	1 tsp. vanilla
8 oz (1 pack) of cream cheese, softened	3/4 c. brown sugar
8 oz. sour cream	

- Mix all but the grapes together in a bowl until smooth. There will be some small chunks
- Stir in washed grapes
- Chill covered and enjoy

SMOKED MAC N' CHEESE

Ingredients	
16 oz. macaroni noodles	8 oz cream cheese cut in chunks
1/4 c. butter	8 oz shredded sharp cheddar
1/4 c. flour	8 oz gouda shredded
3 c. milk	1 c of shredded parmesan cheese
1 tsp salt	
1/2 tsp pepper	

- Preheat smoker to 225 F and make sure wood loaded
- Cook pasta in boiling water to al dente (roughly 7 minutes)
- Melt butter in medium saucepan and whisk in flour once melted, cook and simmer for 2-3 minutes
- Whisk in milk and bring to a boil, cook 5 minutes until thickened
- Stir in cream cheese until smooth and add salt and pepper
- Combine 1 cup of the shredded cheeses, pasta and cream sauce. Spoon into a greased 9x11 pan. Sprinkle top with any remaining cheese
- Place in smoker and cook 1-1.5 hours until brown, bubbly and delicious

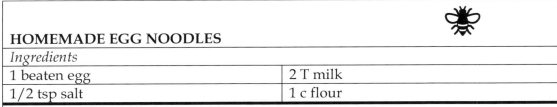

HOMEMADE EGG NOODLES

Ingredients	
1 beaten egg	2 T milk
1/2 tsp salt	1 c flour

- Place flour and salt in bowl and mix.
- Make a "bowl" in the flour and pour egg and milk into it. Mix well.
- Roll out onto counter and let dry for a few hours or overnight
- Once dried, its time to slice. Can either roll it into a roll and slice or use a pizza cutter to cut desired thickness of noodles. (I prefer the latter)

  - Note: I like my noodles about the length of a pinky finger to index finger. When cooked they will become thicker and longer so keep that in mind when deciding thickness and length of noodle
  - Also, if making multiple batches, it works best if no more than 2 batches are made at the same time. If you get too much in the bowl it will not flatten out as nicely and will have worse noodle turnout.

7 LAYER DIP

Ingredients	
1 – 16 oz. can refried beans	1 C shredded lettuce
1 T taco seasoning mix	1 C Mexican style shredded cheese
1 C sour cream	1/2 C green onion slices
1 C salsa	2 T sliced black olives

- Mix beans and taco seasoning. Spread onto the bottom of 9-inch pie pan
- Layer rest of ingredients over the bean mixture (going down and to next column in order)
- Cover and refrigerate.
- Serve with tortilla chips or pita

CINNAMON APPLES

Ingredients	
4 apples peeled and sliced	1/4 tsp nutmeg
1/2 C brown sugar	2 T water
1 tsp cinnamon	1 T butter

- Toss apples, brown sugar, cinnamon and nutmeg in large zip lock bag.
- Cook mixture with remaining ingredients in medium saucepan over medium heat for 8-10 minutes until apples are tender

CHICKEN CAESAR PASTA SALAD

Ingredients

1/2 box of rotini noodles	1 bottle Caesar dressing
1 C shredded parmesan cheese	1 package Caesar croutons
Shredded chicken	Italian seasoning
	Ground black pepper

- Cook rotini pasta in boiling water with 1 T oil added until done. Drain and rinse with cold water.
- Cook 3 chicken breasts and shred. Season with Italian seasoning. If you are running low on time, use 2 large cans of shredded chicken from store.
- Throw pasta in a large bowl, add shredded cheese, dressing (½ to ¾ bottle depending on how much you want) and shredded chicken. Stir together. Season with pepper to taste.
- Cover and chill
- Put croutons in zip lock bag and smash with rolling pin to get smaller chunks. Right before serving, pour over pasta salad and stir together to maintain maximum crispiness of croutons.

FRIED OKRA

Ingredients

Fresh okra	Salt and pepper
buttermilk	cornmeal

- Preheat deep fryer (or begin to warm oil over stove) to 350 F
- Slice okra in approximately ½ - ¾ inch slices
- Soak slices in buttermilk for a few minutes. (milk will start to get a "gummy" thickened texture)
- Place cornmeal in bowl and add desired amount of pepper. Mix well
- Roll okra slices in cornmeal until coated well. (can quickly dip back into buttermilk and roll in cornmeal if you want an extra crispy outside)
- Put coated okra in fryer or in warmed oil for 5-7 minutes.
- Season with salt and enjoy!

GRILLED CHEESE PULL APARTS

Ingredients	
2 cans of refrigerated biscuits (like Pillsbury grands)	3/4 box Velveeta
1/2 C melted butter	

- Preheat oven to 350 F
- Melt butter and pour half into 9-inch round cake pan
- Cut Velveeta into 1-2 inch cubes
- Stuff each biscuit with 1 or 2 cubes of cheese and roll into a ball.
- Arrange dough balls into pan and pour the remaining butter on top
- Plan on larger baking sheet to prevent spilling of cheese.
- Bake for 12 minutes uncovered, then cover in foil and bake for another 12-15 minutes until golden and firm all the way through.
- Cool slightly and enjoy. Goes great with tomato soup or spaghetti-O's.

QUESO DIP

Ingredients	
1 box Velveeta	1 small onion
1 lb. ground beef	Taco seasoning
1 small can of jalapeños	1 to 1.5 tsp Garlic powder
1 small can green chilis	1 T oil
Liquid smoke	

- Brown ground beef, drain and mix with taco seasoning.
- Dice onion into smallest pieces possible. Heat oil over stove in pan. Once hot, add jalapenos, green chilis and onion to pan. Cook completely and add 1-2 shakes of liquid smoke. Stir well.
- Add cheese, beef, garlic powder and half onion mixture to crockpot and melt.
- Once melted, taste test. Add more onion mixture if needed. May also add cumin and chili pepper if not enough of a taco flavor.

ITALIAN ROLLS

Ingredients

1 package Hawaiian rolls	1/4 tsp pepper
Half stick melted butter	1/4 tsp Lawry's all-season salt
1/2 tsp onion powder	Mozzarella cheese
1/2 tsp garlic powder	1 tsp Italian seasoning

- Preheat oven to 400 F
- Separate rolls and put in large zip lock bag
- Add seasoning to bag and pour melted butter over rolls. Shake well to mix all together.
- Add shredded cheese to desired cheesiness and place in baking pan.
- Cook uncovered until cheese is melting.
  - Note: amount of seasoning is by guess, put seasoning in bowl and mix to get desired taste.

BAKING POWDER BISCUITS

Ingredients

2 C flour	3-4 T shortening
3 tsp baking powder	1/2 tsp salt
2/3 to 3/4 C milk	

- Preheat oven to 450 F
- Mix dry ingredients together. Cut shortening into flour mixture.
- Add milk
- Kneed with flour and roll out
- Cut into biscuits and bake on oiled baking pan for 12-15 minutes.

NAAN (LIKE PITA BREAD)

Ingredients	
1 0.25 oz package active dry yeast	1/4 C melted butter
1 C warm water	1 beaten egg
1/4 C sugar	2 tsp salt
3 T milk	4.5 C bread flour (all-purpose will work)
	2 tsp minced garlic, optional

- In bowl, dissolve yeast in warm water and let stand 10 minutes until frothy
- Stir in sugar, milk, egg, salt and enough flour to make soft dough
- Knead 6-8 minutes on lightly floured surface
- Place dough in well oiled bowl and cover with damp cloth. Let rise 1 hour.
- Punch down dough and knead in garlic.
- Pinch off golf ball sized piece of dough and roll into balls. Place on tray and cover with towel to allow to double in size (about 30 minutes)
- During second rising, preheat grill/stove to high heat
- Roll one ball of dough into a thin circle. Lightly oil grill/stove.
- Cook dough 2-3 minutes or until puffy and lightly browned.
- Brush uncooked side with butter and cook until browned (2-4 minutes)
- Repeat with all the dough.

SOUTHERN CORNBREAD

Ingredients	
1 C cornmeal	1/2 C unsalted butter, melted and slightly cooled
1 C flour	1/3 C brown sugar (and dash of white sugar)
1 tsp baking powder	2 T honey
1/2 tsp baking soda	1 large egg
1/8 tsp salt	1 C buttermilk at room temp

- Preheat oven to 400 F. Grease and lightly flour 9-inch square baking pan.
- Whisk cornmeal, flour, baking powder and soda, and salt together in bowl. Set aside
- In another bowl, whisk butter, brown sugar, dash white sugar and honey together until smooth and thick. Whisk in egg until mixed, then add buttermilk and mix.
- Pour wet ingredients into the flour mixture and whisk until combined. Avoid over mixing.
- Pour batter into baking pan and bake for 20 minutes or until golden on top and center cooked through. Use toothpick to test if done.

GRANDMA D'S OLIVE DIP	
Ingredients	
8 oz cream cheese, softened	1/2 tsp dill weed.
1/4 C green olives with pimentos, sliced	

- Once cream cheese softened, add green olives and mix well.
- Add dill weed and mix.
- Cover mixture and refrigerate until chilled.
- Enjoy with crackers

ROSE'S CRISPY POTATOES	
Ingredients	
Potatoes	Salt and pepper
Multiple sticks of butter	

- Preheat oven to 375 F. Slice butter and place several slices on bottom of 9 x 13 pan.
- Slice potatoes as thinly as you can and arrange on bottom and sides of pan. Salt and pepper to liking.
- Add a lot more butter slices on top of this layer and salt/pepper. Repeat layering with butter, potatoes and salt/pepper until desired amount of potatoes used.
- Cover with foil and bake for 1.5-2 hours. The longer you cook, the crispier they will be. Potatoes on side of pan will be brown and crispy like a potato chip.

Entrees

- Mozzarella chicken
- Butter chicken
- Roasted turkey
- Roasted turkey shortened version
- Chicken lasagna
- Puru's chicken curry
- Easy chicken and gravy
- Blackened chicken
- Crispitos
- Tuna bake
- Chicken taco fettucine
- Ham and noodle casserole
- Grandma's beef stroganoff
- Beef tips with gravy
- Matzo ball soup
- Golden rod
- Chicken breasts with cheese
- Jambalaya
- Pot roast
- Chicken Parmesan
- Fried chicken/Chicken strips
- Lasagna
- Bierocks
- Manicotti
- Stuffed pasta shells
- B's chicken and noodles
- Aunt Jenni's famous enchiladas

MOZZARELLA CHICKEN

Ingredients

1 T olive oil	2 T balsamic vinegar
4 boneless skinless chicken breasts	15 oz crushed tomatoes
Salt and pepper	1 T fresh chopped basil
1 T Italian seasoning	Pinch of crushed red pepper flakes
3 cloves garlic	4 slices mozzarella

- In large skillet over medium heat, heat oil. Add chicken and season with salt, pepper and half Italian seasoning. Cook 8 minutes then flip and season the other side. Cook 8 minutes more and set on plate to rest.
- Add garlic to skillet and cook until fragrant (about a minute), then add vinegar to deglaze pan. Scrape up brown bits with wooden spoon, add crushed tomatoes, basil and crushed pepper flakes. Stir well and simmer 10 minutes.
- Return chicken to pan and nestle in sauce. Top chicken with slice of mozzarella and cover with lid until melted.
  - Note: May use a jar of spaghetti sauce if you do not want to use crushed tomatoes.

BUTTER CHICKEN (make Naan to go with it)

Ingredients for marinade:

1/2 C plain yogurt	2 garlic cloves crushed
1 T lemon juice	1.5 lbs. chicken cut into bite sized pieces
1 tsp turmeric powder	*For curry*: 1 T vegetable oil
2 tsp garam masala	1 C tomato sauce
1/2 tsp chili powder or cayenne pepper	1 T sugar
1 tsp cumin	1 1/4 tsp salt
1 T fresh grated ginger	1 cup heavy whipping cream

- For extra smooth sauce combine all marinade ingredients (expect chicken) and blend in food processor (optional step)
- Combine marinade ingredients with chicken in bowl. Cover and refrigerate overnight or up to 24 hours
- Heat vegetable oil over high heat in large fry pan. Add chicken in marinade and cook for 3 minutes or until chicken is white all over.
- Add tomato sauce, sugar and salt. Turn on low and simmer 20 minutes.
- Stir through cream then remove from heat.
- Serve with basmati rice or rice of your choice.

ROASTED TURKEY

Ingredients

1 12-20-pound turkey	2 C kosher salt
1 onion, peeled and quartered	1 C white wine
1 lemon, quartered	*FOR HERB BUTTER:*
Carrots/celery	1 cup unsalted butter, softened
1 bay leaf	1 teaspoon salt
container fresh rosemary	1/2 teaspoon freshly ground black pepper
container fresh thyme	6-8 cloves garlic, minced
Container of fresh sage	fresh chopped herbs

- Rub the turkey inside and out with the salt. Place the bird in a large stock pot, and cover with cold water. Place in the refrigerator and allow the turkey to soak in the salt and water mixture 12 hours, or overnight. I also add ¼ c vinegar and a boat load of ground black pepper and any other seasonings you desire.
- Remove the thawed turkey from the fridge 1 hour before roasting, to let it come to room temperature. Adjust your oven rack so the turkey will sit in the center of the oven
- Preheat oven to 325 degrees F Thoroughly rinse the turkey and discard the brine mixture.
- Make the herb butter by combining room temperature butter, minced garlic, salt, pepper, one tablespoon fresh chopped rosemary, one tablespoon fresh chopped thyme, and half a tablespoon of fresh chopped sage. (You'll use the remaining fresh herbs for stuffing inside the cavity of the turkey)
- Remove turkey from packaging and remove the neck and giblets from the inside the cavities of the bird. (Reserve them for gravy, if you want, or discard them). Pat the turkey very dry with paper towels.
- Season the cavity of the turkey with salt and pepper. Stuff it with the quartered lemon, onion carrots, bay leaf and leftover herbs.
- Use your fingers to loosen and lift the skin above the breasts (on the top of the turkey) and smooth a few tablespoons of the herb butter underneath.
- Tuck the wings of the turkey underneath the turkey and set the turkey on a roasting rack inside a roasting pan (breast side down).
- Microwave the remaining herb butter mixture for 30 seconds (it doesn't need to be completely melted--just really softened). Use a basting brush to brush the remaining herb butter all over the outside of the turkey, legs and wings. Try to leave a little left for later if you can.
- Pour wine and any remaining vegetables in bottom of roasting pan
- Roast at 325 degrees F for about 13-15 minutes per pound (3.5-4 hrs. usually), or until internal temperature (inserted on middle of thigh and breast) reaches about 165 degrees.
- Carefully turn the turkey breast side up about 2/3 through the roasting time, and brush with the remaining butter.
- Allow the bird to stand 20-30 minutes before carving.

ROASTED TURKEY SHORT VERSION

- melt the butter and mix with herbs rather than making an herb butter in this version.
- Rub the turkey inside and out with the kosher salt. Place the bird in a large stock pot, and cover with cold water. Place in the refrigerator and allow the turkey to soak in the salt and water mixture 12 hours, or overnight.
- Preheat oven to 350 degrees F. Thoroughly rinse the turkey and discard the brine mixture.
- Brush the turkey with 1/2 the melted butter. Place breast side down on a roasting rack in a shallow roasting pan. Stuff the turkey cavity with 1 onion, 1/2 the carrots, 1/2 the celery, 1 sprig of thyme, and the bay leaf. Scatter the remaining vegetables and thyme around the bottom of the roasting pan, and cover with the white wine.
- Roast uncovered 3 1/2 to 4 hours in the preheated oven, until the internal temperature of the thigh reaches 165 degrees F. Carefully turn the turkey breast side up about 2/3 through the roasting time, and brush with the remaining butter. Allow the bird to stand about 30 minutes before carving.

CHICKEN LASAGNA

Ingredients

2 C cubed or shredded chicken	1 C parmesan cheese
1 can cream of mushroom soup	8 oz sour cream
1 can cream of chicken soup	1 tsp minced garlic
Lasagna noodles- either no boil or regular	2 C mozzarella and Cheddar cheese, shredded

- Preheat oven to 350 F
- Mix all ingredients together. You may need to add more sour cream or milk to thin it slightly
- If using regular noodles, cook as directed by package. If using no boil noodles, they are ready to use but may not be done all the way after cooking.
- Spread a thin layer or sauce on bottom of 9 x 13 pan. Then layer noodles, chicken mix and cheese. Typically have 3 layers. Make sure shredded cheese is on top.
- Cover with foil and bake for 1 to 1.5 hours. (45 minutes if using already cooked noodles)

PURU'S CHICKEN CURRY

Ingredients (exact amounts were not given)

2-3 T Oil	Turmeric powder
Minced garlic	Cumin
Chopped cilantro	Chili powder
Grated ginger	Curry powder or cubes
One onion	Salt
Chicken cut into bite sized pieces	tomato

- Heat oil with garlic and ginger. Add chopped onion and fry until it starts to brown.
- Add turmeric powder (not much since it makes food bitter) and stir.
- Add chicken pieces and salt. Cook until chicken is done.
- Add cumin, curry powder and chili powder as desired.
- Add some chopped tomatoes, cover pan and let cook for 5-10 minutes. May need to add water.
- May add more curry if needed.
- Serve over rice.
  - Note: I got this recipe from a friend from Nepal. Hands down the best curry I have ever had, but he didn't now know measurements to give. He said it is off taste.

EASY CHICKEN AND GRAVY

Ingredients

Chicken cut into bite sized pieces	Salt/pepper
Butter	Poultry seasoning
Flour	Onion powder
3 C Chicken broth	Garlic powder

- Melt enough butter to generously cover the bottom of a large frying pan. Heat until its barely turning brown.
- Add chicken and season with seasonings. Once chicken is starting to brown, turn it over and cook another minute or two.
- Cover with enough flour to coat chicken well.
- Stir until chicken is well coated, butter is absorbed, and flour starts to cook.
- Add 3 C chicken broth (or enough to cover the chicken)
- Simmer over low heat until chicken is done, and gravy is thickened.
- Serve over rice or mashed potatoes.

BLACKENED CHICKEN

Ingredients

1/4 tsp onion powder	1/4 tsp cayenne pepper
1/4 tsp thyme	1/4 tsp salt
1/4 tsp cumin	1/2 tsp paprika
1/8 tsp white pepper	2 boneless skinless chicken breasts

- Preheat oven to 400 F. Mix spices together. Trim fat from chicken and pat dry.
- Rub olive oil and spices all over chicken.
- Heat cast iron skillet over high heat until smoking (4-5 minutes). Place chicken in skillet and cook 2 min or until crust is formed. Flip and repeat.
- Place chicken in oven on baking sheet until cooked completely.

CRISPITOS

Ingredients

1 lb. ground beef	Tortillas
Taco seasoning	Shredded Mexican cheese blend

- Preheat deep fryer (or oil on stove) to 350 F.
- Cook ground beef, drain and add taco seasoning.
- Put a large spoonful of beef and pinch of shredded cheese onto far side of tortilla and roll up. Use toothpick(s) to keep it rolled together.
- Drop in fryer and cook until tortilla is to desired crispiness (3-5 minutes usually)
- Remove toothpicks and top with shredded cheese.

TUNA BAKE

Ingredients

1/3 c chopped green pepper	1 tsp salt
3 T chopped onion	6 T flour
2 T fat/shortening/butter	1 can chicken with rice soup
1 - 7 oz can tuna	1 1/2 C milk

- Preheat oven to 425 F
- Brown onion and pepper on stove.
- Blend in salt and flour. Add soup and milk. Cook until sauce is thick.
- Add tuna. Pour into greased baking dish.
- Top with baking powder biscuits with grated cheese added.
- Cook 30 minutes.

CHICKEN TACO FETTUCCINE

Ingredients

8 oz uncooked fettuccine	1/2 C heavy whipping cream
2 C cubed cooked chicken	3 – 4 1/2 tsp taco seasoning
1/2 tsp minced garlic	2 T shredded parmesan cheese
1 1/2 tsp olive oil	

- Cook fettucine according to package and drain.
- In large skillet over medium heat cook the chicken and garlic in oil for 4-5 minutes.
- Whisk in cream and taco seasoning until blended.
- Cook and stir until heated through (do not boil)
- Stir in parmesan cheese.
- Toss with fettuccine and serve.

HAM AND NOODLE CASSEROLE

Ingredients

8 oz package of egg noodles cooked	4 T butter
2 C cubed ham	4 T flour
3/4 lb. cheddar cheese	2 C milk
1 can cream of mushroom soup	Cornflake crumbs

- Preheat oven to 350 F
- Cook the butter, flour and milk until thick
- Add cheddar cheese and soup.
- Cook on low until the cheese melts
- Mix with noodles and ham
- Put in 9 x 13 greased pan.
- Sprinkle lightly with cornflake crumbs.
- Bake for 1 hour.

GRANDMA'S BEEF STROGANOFF

Ingredients

1 lb. round steak cut into cubes	1 can cream of mushroom soup
2 T fat	1 can tomato soup
1/2 C onion	1/2 tsp salt
flour	

- Put everything together and simmer for 1 hour.
- Serve over noodles, spaghetti, or rice.

BEEF TIPS WITH GRAVY

Ingredients

2 lbs beef tenderloin, stew meat or roast	1 packet brown gravy
1 can cream of mushroom soup	1 packet onion soup mix
1.5 C water	4 oz can of mushrooms (optional)

- Preheat oven to 300 F. Add cubed meat to 9 x 13 pan.
- In large bowl, mix remaining ingredients and pour over meat.
- Add mushrooms and stir to coat.
- Cover with foil and bake for 2.5 -3 hours.
- Serve over rice, mashed potatoes, or egg noodles.

MATZO BALL SOUP

Ingredients

6 C chicken stock	1 C matzo meal
1 carrot	1/4 C chicken stock
1 rib celery	4 eggs separated
1/2 onion chopped	1/4 C vegetable oil
1/4 C parsley	

- Combine ingredients in left column and bring to a boil. Reduce heat and simmer until veggies are tender.
- Combine all but egg whites and mix. In a separate bowl beat egg whites until frothy but not stiff.
- Fold into rest of ingredients and refrigerate for 15 minutes.
- Form into balls and drop into simmering soup. Cover and cook for 30 minutes.
  - Note: dip hands into water occasionally while making balls.

GOLDEN ROD

Ingredients

4-6 hardboiled eggs	Milk to cover
cornstarch	

- Slice eggs and cover with milk. Salt and pepper to season.
- Heat and add cornstarch to thicken.
- Serve over toast

CHICKEN BREASTS WITH CHEESE

Ingredients

4 boneless chicken breasts	1 package Monterrey jack cheese
flour	

- Cut cheese into a smaller blocks.
- Wrap chicken around the cheese and use toothpick to hold together.
- Refrigerate overnight.
- Roll breasts in flour and brown on stove.
- Place on cookie sheet and bake at 425 F until cheese melts (about 10-15 minutes)

JAMBALAYA

Ingredients

1 box jambalaya mix	2-3 chicken breasts
3 C chicken broth	Andouille sausage

- Add garlic powder, onion powder, black pepper, and Cajun seasoning to chicken broth. Bring to a boil and cook chicken in boiling broth.
- Once chicken is done, shred it.
- Make jambalaya according to package directions but use the chicken broth instead of water. Add the chicken and sausage.
- Enjoy

POT ROAST

Ingredients

1 beef or pork roast	1 can golden mushroom soup
Bay leaf	1 jar or brown gravy
Sage, thyme, rosemary, pepper, Lawry's, onion and garlic	potatoes
Sliced carrots	Beef broth

- Preheat oven to 350 F
- Season roast with seasonings and sear all sides on hot frying pan.
- Place roast in roasting pan and add beef broth to top of roast. Add bay leaf.
- Cook for 3 hours.
- Remove roast. Slice potatoes and carrots. Add to roast. Pour brown gravy and golden mushroom soup over roast and potatoes.
- Cook for another hour or until potatoes are done.

CHICKEN PARMESAN

Ingredients

Boneless skinless chicken breasts	1 jar regular pasta sauce
2 eggs, beaten	1 jar vodka sauce
Spaghetti noodles, cooked	1 C flour
1/4 tsp garlic powder, onion powder, Lawry's,	1/2 tsp black pepper, Italian seasoning, parmesan cheese grated
1/2 C Italian breadcrumbs	1/2 C milk/buttermilk
Sliced mozzarella cheese	

- Preheat oven to 375 F
- Mix milk and eggs together. In a separate bowl, mix seasonings, breadcrumbs and flour. (may need to adjust seasoning amounts to taste, these are conservative amounts)
- Dip the chicken into the egg mix and then dip in flour mix to cover well. If you want an extra crispy chicken, repeat this step
- Fry chicken either on the stove in oil or in deep fryer for 2-3 minutes each side.
- Place on baking sheet and bake until cooked all the way.
- Mix the jars of pasta sauce and heat over stove.
- The last few minutes of cook time, place small amount of sauce on chicken and cheese slice over this and melt in oven.
- Put cooked spaghetti on bottom of plate, pasta, chicken breast and sauce over this, if you like.

FRIED CHICKEN/CHICKEN STRIPS

Ingredients

For brine: 8 C water, 1/2 C kosher salt, ¼ C honey, 1 T black peppercorns, 1 lemon halved, 1 head garlic, 3 bay leaves, 6 sprigs of thyme	For coating: 3 C flour, 2 T garlic powder, 2 T onion powder, 2 tsp paprika, 2 tsp cayenne pepper, 2 tsp Lawry's, 1/2 tsp black pepper, 1/2 tsp poultry seasoning
2 C buttermilk with 1 tsp salt and 1/2 tsp black pepper and 1 egg	Chicken pieces of your desire (legs, wings, etc.) or tenderloins if doing strips

- In a large pot combine brine ingredients and bring to boil. Boil for 1 minute and stir to dissolve salt. Remove from heat and cool completely.
- Add chicken to cooled brine and refrigerate for 12 hours
- Remove chicken from brine and rinse clean. Pat dry.
- Let chicken rest for 1.5 hours or until it comes to room temp.
- Add oil to a large pot at least 2 inches high but no more than 1/3 up the side of the pan.
- Combine coating ingredients in large bowl. Place buttermilk with salt/pepper in separate bowl.
- Dip the chicken into the milk mixture and then into flour mix. May repeat if desire extra crispy chicken.
- Heat oil to 320 F, drop a few pieces of chicken at a time into oil and cook until deep golden brown and cooked through. (7-12 minutes). Fry breasts at 340 F if bone in.
  - Note: do not overcrowd the chicken in pan or it will not cook as well. Do not try to rush chicken and turn up heat or you will have burnt chicken.

BIEROCKS

Ingredients

1 bag Rhode's frozen rolls, Texas sized	2 lbs. ground beef, cooked, drained and seasoned
Cabbage, shredded thin	Onion, optional

- Grease cookie sheet with Crisco. Lightly grease each frozen roll and set on cookie sheet 2-3 inches apart. Let rise to room temp with tea towel covering pan. Rolls should be about the size of them after cooking.
- Lay wax paper on baking sheet and lightly flour it. Flatten each roll and pull them with hands to make large rectangles.
- Brown the ground beef and season as desired. Add shredded cabbage and onion, if using, to ground beef. Cover and let simmer 20-30 minutes until cabbage is transparent. Stirring occasionally. Let mix cool slightly.
- Scoop meat mix onto flat dough and fold dough over stuffing. Place fold down on baking sheet and bake at 350 F until golden brown.

LASAGNA

Ingredients	
Lasagna noodles cooked	1 jar spaghetti sauce
Shredded mozzarella cheese	1 lb. ground beef
1tsp Italian seasoning	1/4 tsp garlic powder, onion powder, Lawry's
Pinch of brown sugar	

- Preheat oven to 425 F
- Brown ground beef and drain. Mix in seasonings and brown sugar.
- Add meat to the spaghetti sauce and mix
- Put small amount of sauce on bottom of 9 x 13 pan.
- Add lasagna noodles side by side (usually 3 wide to fill pan)
- Top with sauce mix and shredded cheese.
- Repeat until pan filled (usually 3 layers) and top with plenty of shredded cheese. I also usually put some shredded cheddar on top as well for looks. Sprinkle top with Italian seasoning.
- Cover and bake in oven for 30 minutes or until cheese melted

MANICOTTI

Ingredients	
1 pint ricotta cheese	3/4 C grated parmesan cheese
8 oz shredded mozzarella cheese	2 eggs
1 tsp parsley	Salt and pepper to taste
1 jar spaghetti sauce	Manicotti pasta, cooked

- Preheat oven to 350 F
- In large bowl, combine ricotta, mozzarella and 1/2 C parmesan, eggs, parsley and salt/pepper. Mix well.
- Pour sauce in bottom of 9 x 13 pan to lightly cover bottom.
- Fill each manicotti shell with cheese mixture (usually about 3 Tbs.) and arrange in pan.
- Pour remaining sauce over pasta, sprinkle with remaining parmesan.
- Bake 45 minutes or until bubbly

STUFFED PASTA SHELLS (make with Italian rolls)

Ingredients

1 lb. ground beef	Pasta shell noodles, cooked
Mozzarella cheese, shredded	Lawry's, garlic powder, onion powder, Italian seasoning to taste
1 jar spaghetti sauce	

- Preheat oven to 400 F
- In bottom of 9x13 pan pour some sauce to cover bottom.
- Rinse cooked pasta shells in cold water to easier handling.
- Brown ground beef, drain and season to taste. Mix with spaghetti sauce.
- Stuff each shell with desired amount of meat and sauce mixture. Arrange in pan.
- Cover with the shredded mozzarella cheese
- Bake 15-20 minutes or until cheese is slightly browned.

B's CHICKEN AND NOODLES

Ingredients

Egg noodles (homemade or Reame's)	3-4 boneless, skinless chicken breasts
Carrots and celery, sliced	1 small onion, diced (can use onion powder)
1 tsp Lawry's	1/2 tsp turmeric
1/4 tsp white pepper	1/2 to 1 tsp black pepper
1-1.5 tsp poultry seasoning	1 tsp garlic powder or minced garlic
Chicken broth/bouillon	1 bay leaf
1 dash liquid smoke	

- Fill stock pot 1/2 to 3/4 full of chicken broth, liquid smoke, bay leaf, and seasonings. Bring to a boil. Either canned broth or bouillon. I add an extra bouillon cube or two to give broth a stronger flavor.
- Add chicken to broth and cook for 10-15 minutes. Remove chicken and shred it. Set aside.
- Add the vegetables to broth and simmer 10 minutes.
- Increase heat to medium (6-7 setting on my stove) and add noodles. Cook for 10 minutes.
- Add chicken back to broth and simmer for roughly 5 minutes to ensure noodles are cooked through.
- If broth is not thick enough, mix 3 T flour with a little water and stir until smooth. Pour this into broth and simmer for 5 minutes. This will thicken. Repeat if needed.
- Serve over mashed potatoes.
  - Note: this is the shortcut version rather than boiling bone-in chicken in water for hours. This is also a rough estimate of seasoning amounts, they will need to be adjusted to your taste and preference. To make soup, simply increase the amount of broth.

AUNT JENNI'S FAMOUS ENCHILADAS

Ingredients	
Cheddar cheese, shredded (by hand is best)	2-2.5 lbs. ground beef
Bag of dried chili pepper "pods"	Flour tortillas (Mama Lupe's best), medium sized
Seasoning for meat	3-4 whole cloves

- Tear off end and stem from chili pods, cut open and remove all seeds. Rinse thoroughly. Place chilis in pot and cover with water. Boil until water is dark and chilis are soft and rehydrated. Dump most of water off and place in a blender with 3-4 whole cloves
- Blend with a small amount of water until pureed. This is your enchilada sauce so the thinner, the better. Take a small amount on your finger and taste, if too hot, add some water and repeat.
- Warm tortillas until brown on both sides on stove burner. Do a few at a time and place between a tea towel to keep them warm and pliable.
- Brown meat and season as desired.
- Pour some sauce in bottom of 9x13 pan. Dip tortillas in sauce and place on cookie sheet. (your sauce will gradually get thicker with the more tortillas you use). Place a handful of meat and cheese on tortilla and roll up leaving ends open. Use hand to apply small amount of sauce on each rolled up enchilada. Can either freeze them at this step or continue to cook.
- Warm an electric griddle and oil it. Once oil heated, place fold down on griddle and fry until browned. Flip over and repeat until meat and cheese warmed and melted. Sprinkle more cheese on top.
  - Note: Jenni's tips for success- never touch canned enchilada sauce and authentic enchiladas are fried, not cooked in the oven. Hand shredded cheese melts better and is less waxy. Color of enchilada sauce should be a nice red- think cayenne pepper to chili powder color.

CROCKPOT

- Shredded BBQ pork
- Bacon chicken chili
- Chili
- French dips
- Peach cobbler
- Chicken and dumplings
- Enchiladas
- Lasagna soup
- Pork loin with gravy
- Ranch and onion whole chicken
- Chicken and rice
- Beef stew
- Shredded BBQ pork

SHREDDED BBQ PORK

Ingredients

1 pork loin or roast	1 jar BBQ sauce
Hamburger buns or desired bun	BBQ seasoning of choice

- Generously cover pork with BBQ seasoning and sear all sides.
- Place in crock pot and cover in BBQ sauce.
- Cook on high for 6-8 hours or until tender and falls apart easily
- Shred pork using forks or electric mixer
- Place on buns and enjoy

BACON CHICKEN CHILI

Ingredients

4 oz can green chilis	2 cans white chili beans
Roughly 6 strips cooked bacon	1 can chicken broth
1 lb. chicken breasts, shredded	1 can cream of chicken soup
1 medium onion, diced	2 limes
2 tsp oregano, garlic powder and cumin	1.5 tsp coriander
1 tsp chili powder	1/2 tsp paprika, white pepper
Black pepper to taste	3 T olive oil

- Cook diced onion in 3 T olive oil until transparent. Add green chilis and cook for 5 minutes. I also add 1 shake of liquid smoke for a smokier flavor.
- Add everything but the limes to the crockpot and stir together well.
- Add black pepper to taste.
- Cook on high for 3-4 hours or low for 6-8 hours.
- Squeeze limes into chili roughly 15 minutes prior to serving.

BEEF CHILI

Ingredients

1 lb. ground beef	1 can chili beans
Chili seasoning	Tomato sauce

- Brown beef and drain well. Mix with chili seasoning.
- Add beef and beans, undrained, to crockpot.
- Add tomato sauce until desired consistency. Keep in mind it will thicken up as it cooks.
- Cook on high for 4 hours or low for 8 hours.

FRENCH DIPS

Ingredients

Hoagie buns	1 beef roast
Beef broth	1 package dry onion soup mix
1 package au jus	1 bay leaf
1 tsp sage, garlic powder, Lawry's	1.5 tsp black pepper
Sliced provolone cheese	

- Mix seasonings together and rub roast. Sear all sides.
- Put roast in crockpot. Add bay leaf. Sprinkle onion soup mix over roast.
- Pour beef broth over roast to 3/4 the way up the roast.
- Cook on high for 4-5 hours or low for 8 hours. Shred meat.
- Make au jus according to package directions or can use drippings from crockpot as au jus.
- Place sliced provolone on bun and add desired amount of shredded meat.
- Dip sandwich into au jus and enjoy!

PEACH COBBLER

Ingredients

3/4 C Bisquick baking mix	1/3 C sugar
1/2 C brown sugar	1/2 can evaporated milk
2 tsp melted butter	2 large eggs
3 large ripe peaches, mashed	2 tsp vanilla
3/4 tsp cinnamon	

- Lightly grease crockpot with spray
- In large bowl, combine sugar and baking mix. Add eggs and vanilla, mix well.
- Add butter and milk, stir together.
- Mix in peaches and cinnamon until well mixed.
- Pour into crockpot.
- Cook on low 6-8 hours or high 3-4 hours.
- Serve warm and with ice cream.

CHICKEN AND DUMPLINGS

Ingredients

4 chicken breasts	1 small onion
2 T butter	1-2 can biscuit dough, cut into pieces
2 cans cream of chicken soup	8 to 10 oz chicken broth
1 tsp black pepper, onion powder, garlic powder, poultry seasoning, Lawry's	

- Season chicken and place in crockpot with butter, soup and onion. Fill with broth to cover chicken.
- Cook on low 8 hours or high 5-6 hours.
- Shred chicken and stir well.
- Add pieces of dough 1.5-2 hours prior to serving.

ENCHILADAS

Ingredients

Pork or chicken, whichever desired	Tortillas
Shredded cheese of your choosing	1-2 large cans of Red enchilada sauce
Taco seasoning	

- Season meat and place in crockpot. Cover with enchilada sauce.
- Cook on high 4-5 hours and low 6-8.
- Remove meat and shred. Preheat oven to 400 F
- Pour some of the sauce in crockpot into bottom of 9x13 pan.
- Spoon shredded meat into tortilla with some shredded cheese. Roll together and place in pan. Repeat until pan filled.
- Pour enchilada sauce from crockpot over enchiladas. Top with shredded cheese.
- Bake until cheese is melted.

LASAGNA SOUP

Ingredients

1 T oil	1 diced onion
1 T chopped garlic	2 lbs. ground beef
1 T Italian seasoning	2 tsp pepper, salt
1 jar pasta sauce	4 C beef broth
1 can crushed tomatoes (optional)	12 oz Mafalda noodles or lasagna noodles broken up
1/2 C heavy cream	1 cup mozzarella cheese, shredded
1 C jack cheese blend, shredded	

- Heat oil on stove and cook onion until translucent. Add garlic and cook 1 minute.
- Add browned ground beef and sprinkle with seasonings.
- Add everything but the cream and cheeses to crockpot and stir.
- Cook on high for 4 hours or low 6-8 hours.
- Add the heavy cream and cheeses, stir and enjoy.

PORK LOIN WITH GRAVY

Ingredients

1 pork loin	1 can cream of mushroom soup
1 pork gravy mix	1/2 C water

- Place loin in crockpot. Spoon soup over loin and sprinkle gravy mix evenly over everything.
- Pour water to the top of loin.
- Cook on low 5-6 hours.
- Place loin on serving dish and pour gravy from crockpot over it.
- Serve with mashed potatoes or rice.

RANCH ONION CHICKEN

Ingredients

5 lb. whole chicken	1 dry onion soup mix
1 dry ranch mix	3 garlic cloves crushed and peeled
1 tsp paprika and black pepper	1/2 tsp Lawry's

- Add ranch and onion soup mixes and seasonings to bowl, mix well.
- Rinse chicken, remove innards and pat dry.
- Generously rub seasoning mix to inside and outside of chicken. Place garlic inside chicken. Place in zip-lock bag overnight to marinate (optional step)
- Place chicken into crockpot.
- Cook on high 4 hours or low for 8 hours. Make sure the thick part of the breast is 165 F.

CHICKEN AND RICE

Ingredients

1 box Zatarain's yellow rice, cooked	4 chicken breasts
2 C shredded cheddar cheese	1 medium onion diced
1 can cream of chicken soup	1 can corn, drained
1.5 C chicken stock	Poultry seasoning, salt, pepper

- Place chicken in crockpot and season to your liking. Sprinkle onions on top.
- Mix chicken broth and can of soup together.
- Pour over chicken
- Cook on low 7-8 hours or high for 4 hours.
- Shred chicken right before serving and add cooked rice, cheese and corn.
- Stir and cook until cheese is melted.
- Serve warm.

CHEESEBURGER SOUP

Ingredients

4 small potatoes, peeled and diced	1 small onion, diced
1 c shredded carrots	1/2 C cut celery
1 tsp basil	1 tsp parsley
3 C chicken broth	1 lb. ground beef
3 T butter	1/4 C flour
2 C milk	1/2 tsp each of salt and pepper
1 package Velveeta, cubed or 2 C shredded cheddar cheese	

- Place potatoes, onions, carrots, celery, basil and parsley in crockpot. Pour chicken broth over.
- Cook on low 6-8 hours or high 4-5 hours.
- 45 minutes prior to serving, brown ground beef and drain. Add to crockpot.
- Melt butter in skillet. Whisk in flour and cook until golden brown and bubbly (1 minute). Whisk in milk and salt/pepper. Pour into crockpot and stir.
- Add cheese to crockpot and cook until cheese in melted. Roughly 30 minutes.

BEEF STEW

Ingredients

1/4 C flour	Boneless beef roast, cut into 1-inch cubes
2 T vegetable oil	1.5-2.5 C water
2 beef bouillon cubes	1 can tomato soup
3 tsp Italian seasoning	2 bay leaves
1.5 tsp pepper	1 large onion, sliced
2-3 large russet potatoes, peeled and cut into 1.5-inch pieces.	2 carrots and stalks of celery, sliced
Can of drained mushrooms and peas (optional)	

- Pour flour into 1-gallon zip lock bag, add meat and shake to evenly coat.
- Add oil to large skillet and heat. Brown meat in batches and add to crockpot.
- Add water and bouillon cubes to skillet and cook. Ensure you get the brown pieces at bottom of pan mixed with bouillon. Once mixed well, remove from heat and add tomato soup, Italian seasoning, bay leaves, and pepper. Stir.
- Pour into crockpot over beef. Add onions, potatoes, carrots, celery and mushrooms/peas, if using.
- Cook on low for 8 hours or until beef/veggies are very tender. Add water if needed.

Baked Goods

- Salted nut roll cake
- Sopapilla cheesecake
- Lemonade cake
- "To die for" brownies
- B's butter cake
- Pecan pie
- Monkey bread
- No bake cookies
- Fudge filled cheesecake
- Better than sex cake
- Banana bars
- Grandma D's chocolate cake
- No name candy
- Banana bread
- Caramels
- Oreo balls
- Hard candy
- Oatmeal scotchies
- Easy fudge
- Puppy chow
- Chewy brownies
- Malted pretzel crunch
- Apple pie bites
- Christmas crack
- Gorp
- Molasses cookies
- Heidi's cream cheese bars
- Perfect rice krispie bars
- Molten lava cakes
- Fruity pebble cheesecake bites
- 1-hour cinnamon rolls
- Cream cheese cinnamon roll frosting
- Aunt Jenni's monster cookies

SALTED NUT ROLL CAKE

Ingredients

1 box yellow cake mix	1 egg
3/4 C melted butter	3 C mini marshmallows
12 oz peanut butter chips	1/2 C corn syrup
1 tsp vanilla	2 C peanuts
2 C Rice Krispies	

- Preheat oven to 350 F
- Mix cake mix, egg and 1/4 C butter. Press into greased 9x13 pan. Bake for 10-12 minutes.
- Place marshmallows on top and bake until marshmallows are puffed up, about 3-5 minutes.
- Melt peanut butter chips, corn syrup and 1/2 C butter over stove. Stir in vanilla.
- Add rice krispies and peanuts, stirring to mix well.
- Pour over marshmallows and chill.
- Slice into portions before it gets too hard.

SOPAPILLA CHEESECAKE

Ingredients

2 cans butter crescent rolls	2 packages cream cheese, softened
1 cup sugar	1 tsp vanilla
1/4 C melted butter	1 T cinnamon
1/4 C sugar	1/4 C brown sugar

- Preheat oven to 350 F.
- Combine cream cheese, 1 cup sugar and vanilla until smooth.
- Press one can of crescent rolls into bottom of 9x13 pan. Spread cheesecake mixture on bottom layer and top with second can of crescent rolls.
- Combine cinnamon, 1/4 C sugar and brown sugar. Pour melted butter over top and sprinkle cinnamon sugar mixture.
- Cook 30 minutes

LEMONADE CAKE

Ingredients

For cake: 1 box lemon cake mix	*For glaze*: 2 C powdered sugar
1 box instant lemon pudding	1/2 C lemonade mix (regular or strawberry lemonade)
4 eggs	1/2 C water
1 C water	2 T melted butter
1/2 C oil	

- Preheat oven to 350 F. Mix all ingredients for cake together in bowl.
- Bake in greased pan for 30 minutes or until done.
- Mix glaze after cake comes out of oven.
- Poke holes in cake 5 minutes after it comes out of the oven, then pour glaze over cake (it will look like a lot of glaze).
- Lift edged of cake to allow glaze to cover bottom of cake.
- Cool completely and enjoy.

"TO DIE FOR "BROWNIES

Ingredients

For cake: 1 bod chocolate cake mix (devil's food is awesome)	*For caramel filling*: 1 11 oz bag of caramels unwrapped
1 C evaporated milk	1/3 C evaporated milk
1 stick melted butter	
2 C chocolate chips (milk or semi-sweet)	

- Preheat oven to 350 F.
- Grease 9x13 pan.
- In medium bowl, combine cake mix, 1 C evap. Milk and melted butter. Mix well and batter will be thick.
- Spread half of batter on bottom of pan and bake for 15 minutes.
- Start caramel filling while bottom is baking. Over medium heat, melt caramels and evap. Milk. Stir frequently until melted and smooth.
- When bottom is done baking (only partially cooked), take out of oven and sprinkle with 2 C of chocolate chips then drizzle caramel sauce over the whole thing.
- Drop the rest of the batter and drop by teaspoonfuls onto caramel layer.
- Bake for another 25-30 minutes until center is set.

B's BUTTER CAKE

Ingredients

For cake: 1 box yellow or butter cake mix	For crust: 1/4 C melted butter
3/4 C melted butter	1 package cream cheese, softened
2 eggs	2 eggs
1 tsp vanilla	1 tsp vanilla
	2-3 C powdered sugar

- Preheat oven to 350 F.
- Mix ingredients for cake. Pat into bottom of 9x13 pan with fingers.
- Mix cream cheese, 2 eggs, 1/4 C melted butter, and vanilla with an electric beater. Slowly mix in the powdered sugar. Pour over cake layer.
- Bake for 40-45 minutes.
- Sprinkle powdered sugar over top or raspberry ice cream topping.
- Best served warm and with ice cream.

PECAN PIE

Ingredients

1/4 C brown sugar	1 C sugar
1 9-inch-deep dish pie crust (I use refrigerated in the biscuit aisle)	1 C light corn syrup
1.5 tsp vanilla	1/2 tsp salt
1/8 tsp cinnamon	4 eggs, beaten
1 stick salted butter	2 C pecans (plus extra for top if desired)
Dash of nutmeg	

- Partially pre-bake a 9-inch pie crust after using fork to poke holes in crust (6-8 minutes at 400 F until bottom just beginning to color). Then preheat oven to 350 F.
- Melt butter in saucepan over medium heat. Add brown sugar and whisk until smooth. Remove from heat and add sugar, corn syrup, vanilla, and salt. Mix well.
- Add beaten eggs to mixture and stir well.
- Stir in pecans and pour into pie crust.
- Bake for 50-60 minutes on baking sheet until filling is set (slightly jiggly but not sloshy). Once filling set, let cool completely before slicing.

MONKEY BREAD

Ingredients

2/3 C sugar	4 tubes of biscuits of your choice
1 tsp cinnamon	1.5 sticks butter
1 C brown sugar	

- Preheat oven to 350 F.
- Mix sugar and cinnamon and place in a plastic bag.
- Cut each biscuit into 4's. Form into balls. Grease bundt pan.
- Coat each ball of dough with cinnamon sugar and arrange in pan.
- Melt butter and brown sugar together. Pour over dough balls.
- Bake for 30 minutes. Let cool for 10 minutes before turning over onto plate.

NO BAKE COOKIES

Ingredients

2 C sugar	6 T cocoa
Pinch of salt	1/2 C butter
1/2 C milk	1 tsp vanilla
3 C instant oatmeal	

- Mix everything but vanilla and oatmeal in saucepan and let boil for 3 minutes.
- Add the vanilla and instant oatmeal. Form into balls and put on waxed paper to cool.

FUDGE FILLED CHEESECAKE

Ingredients

4- 8 oz cream cheese	4 large eggs
1.5 C sugar	12 oz semisweet or milk chocolate chips
Whipped cream-optional	1 premade graham cracker pie crust

- Beat cream cheese at medium speed with electric mixer until light and fluffy. Gradually add sugar and beat well.
- Add eggs one at a time, beating just until yellow disappears. Stir in vanilla but don't overmix.
- Pour half of batter into crust. Sprinkle with chocolate chips to withing 3/4 inch of edge. Pour in remaining batter starting at outer edge and working towards center.
- Place on baking sheet and bake for 1 hour or until set. Cool on rack 1 hour.
- Serve slightly warm. May garnish with whipped cream or chocolate shavings.

BETTER THAN SEX CAKE

Ingredients

1 box chocolate cake mix (devil's food or German chocolate)	1 can sweetened condensed milk
1 container whipped cream	1 jar caramel ice cream topping
2-3 Heath bars, crushed	

- Preheat oven to temp indicated on box and make cake according to directions.
- Once cake removed from oven, let cool slightly and poke holes all over cake.
- Mix sweetened cond. Milk and caramel filling together well. Pour over cake.
- Spread whipped cream over top of cake. Sprinkle with crushed heath bars.
- Cool and enjoy!

BANANA BARS

Ingredients

1/2 C butter, softened	Dash of salt
2 C sugar	1 tsp baking soda
3 eggs	For frosting: 1 package cream cheese, softened
1.5 C mashed bananas (about 3 bananas)	4 C powdered sugar
1 tsp vanilla	2 tsp vanilla
2 C flour	1/2 C butter

- Preheat oven to 350 F. Cream butter and sugar until light and fluffy.
- Beat eggs, bananas and vanilla into mix.
- Stir dry ingredients in until blended. Pour into a greased 15x10 baking sheet.
- Bake for 20-25 minutes.
- Brown 1/2 C butter with a pinch of brown sugar. Let cool then beat cream cheese and butter together until fluffy. Add vanilla and powdered sugar.
- Frost bars and enjoy.

GRANDMA D's CHOCOLATE CAKE

Ingredients

For cake: 1/2 C butter	*For topping*: 1 C sugar
1 C sugar	1/3 C evaporated milk
4 eggs	1 stick butter
16 oz chocolate syrup	1/2 C semi-sweet chocolate chips
1/8 tsp salt	1 tsp vanilla
1 tsp baking powder	
1 C flour	

- Mix ingredients for cake adding eggs 1 at a time. Bake at 350 F for 25-30 minutes in a 9x13 pan.
- Melt together ingredients for topping and pour over cake.

NO NAME CANDY

Ingredients

2 bags chocolate chips	1 C butter
2 bags butterscotch chips	2 lbs. powdered sugar
2 bags peanut butter chips	1 package instant vanilla pudding
	1/2 C milk
	1 tsp maple flavoring

- Melt together 1 bag of each of the chips and pour into a greased 10x15 pan. Let set.
- Beat ingredients in right column together and spread over chocolate mixture. Let set.
- Repeat step one with remaining chips and pour over top. Let set.

BANANA BREAD

Ingredients

1 1/4 C sugar	1 tsp baking soda
1/2 C shortening/butter	1/2 tsp salt
2 eggs	1/4 C sour milk/buttermilk
2 C flour, sifted	3 mashed bananas

- Preheat oven to 325 F. Cream butter and sugar together.
- Add eggs and cream until light. Sift flour, soda and salt. Add alternately with sour milk and bananas mixed together.
- In greased and floured loaf pan, bake for 60-70 minutes.

CARAMELS

Ingredients

1 can sweetened condensed milk	2 1/4 C brown sugar
1 C light corn syrup	1 C butter
1 tsp vanilla	

- Put everything together in saucepan and bring to a boil. Stir constantly until temp is 235 F.
- Pour in greased bar pan. The bigger the pan, the thinner the easier to cut.
- When cool, cut up and wrap in wax paper or eat right out of pan.

OREO BALLS

Ingredients

1 package oreos, crushed	White almond bark
1 8 oz package of cream cheese, softened	

- Mix oreos and cream cheese.
- Roll into walnut sized balls and chill for an hour on baking sheet.
- Melt white almond bark, dip balls into bark with toothpick.
- Harden on wax paper.

HARD CANDY

Ingredients

2 C light corn syrup	2 C sugar
1 tsp flavoring oil (strawberry, butterscotch, etc.)	6 drops food coloring

- In heavy saucepan with deep sides, combine syrup and sugar. Boil to a hard crack (300-350 F).
- Remove from heat and add flavor oil. Add coloring.
- Pour into well oiled baking sheet. Cool enough to score candy with knife. Score for easier breakup. Cool completely and break apart. Will be in "shards" more than pretty squares.

OATMEAL SCOTCIHIES

Ingredients

1 batch oatmeal cookies or package	Butterscotch chips
White chocolate chips	

- Make your favorite oatmeal cookie recipe or a store-bought package.
- Prior to putting in oven, add half bag of butterscotch chips and white chocolate chips to batter and mix well.
- Scoop cookies onto baking sheet as normal and bake as directed.

EASY FUDGE

Ingredients

3 C chocolate chips	1 tsp vanilla
14 oz sweetened cond. Milk	1/4 tsp salt
1/4 C (4T) butter	

- Line pan with aluminum foil or parchment paper.
- Combine chips, butter and sw. cond. Milk. Microwave in 1-minute increments until melted (2-3 minutes) or melt together over stove.
- Stir and add vanilla and salt.
- Pour in pan and chill in fridge for 2 hours.
  - Note: this is much less labor intensive but tastes just as good, if not better than the time-consuming fudges.

PUPPY CHOW

Ingredients

12 oz chocolate chips	1/2 C peanut butter
1 lb. powdered sugar	1 box rice or corn Chex

- Melt chocolate chips with peanut butter.
- Pour cereal in large bowl and pour the chocolate mix over. Mix well.
- In paper sack, add half the powdered sugar. Pour in cereal mix and top with rest of powdered sugar.
- Shake to coat well.
- Enjoy!

CHEWY BROWNIES

Ingredients

3/4 C cocoa	2.5 sticks butter
2 C sugar	1 C flour
4 eggs, beaten	2 tsp vanilla
1 C nuts, optional	

- Preheat oven to 325 F.
- Melt together butter and cocoa. Blend flour and sugar into mixture.
- Beat in the eggs and vanilla.
- Cook in greased 9x13 pan for 35 minutes.

MALTED PRETZEL CRUNCH

Ingredients

4 C salted mini pretzels	1/2 C packed brown sugar
1/4 C sugar	6 T milk powder
1/4 C malted milk powder	1/2 tsp salt, optional
14 T butter, melted	

- Preheat oven to 275 F.
- Crush pretzels in a Ziplock bag to 1/4 their original size.
- Add the milk powder, malt powder, sugar, brown sugar and salt. Toss to mix.
- Pour butter over mix and shake to coat.
- Spread clusters on parchment paper and bake for 20 minutes or until toasted.
- Cool completely before storing or easing.

APPLE PIE BITES

Ingredients

1 granny smith apple	1 can crescent rolls
1 tsp apple pie spice	3 T butter
1/4 C brown sugar	

- Preheat oven to 375 F.
- Place crescent rolls flat on tray lines with parchment paper. Slice apple.
- Spread brown sugar and apple pie spice over rolls.
- Roll apple slice into butter and place on wide end of crescent. Roll crescent roll up.
- Bake 10-12 minutes.

CHRISTMAS CRACK

Ingredients

About 1 sleeve of saltine crackers	1 C dark brown sugar
1 C unsalted butter	1/4 tsp salt
1 tsp vanilla	2 C chocolate chips of your choice

- Preheat oven to 400 F. Line 10x15 pan with aluminum foil. Spray with baking spray.
- Line with saltines in a single layer on bottom to completely cover bottom.
- Place brown sugar, butter and salt in saucepan. Cook on medium heat, stirring frequently until butter melts. Continue to cook 3-5 minutes until mix comes to a boil and starts to darken. Remove from heat and stir in vanilla.
- Pour brown sugar mixture over crackers and spread evenly. Bake 5 minutes.
- Microwave chocolate chips in 30 second intervals until melted. Stir each time.
- Once caramel is no longer bubbling, pour melted chocolate over crackers and spread evenly on top.
- Cool to room temp then place in fridge overnight.
- Remove foil from bottom of candy and cut into snack sized pieces with chef knife.

GORP

Ingredients

1 1/3 C sugar	1 C butter
1/2 C light corn syrup	6-7 C rice Chex
Peanuts, M&M's, optional	2 tsp vanilla

- Boil sugar, butter and corn syrup to soft ball stage (235-245 F). Add vanilla and peanuts, if desired.
- Pour over 6-7 C Chex cereal in paper bag. Shake to coat well. Add M&Ms and shake again.
- Spread onto waxed paper to cool.

MOLASSES COOKIES

Ingredients

3/4 C butter, melted	2 C flour
1 C sugar	2 tsp baking soda
1 egg	1/2 tsp salt
1/4 C molasses	1 tsp cinnamon
1/2 tsp cloves	1/2 tsp ginger

- Mix butter, sugar, egg, and mix until smooth. Add molasses.
- In a separate bowl, mix dry ingredients and add to molasses mix.
- Chill covered for 1 hour in fridge.
- Preheat oven to 375 F. Roll dough into balls and roll in sugar.
- Bake 8-10 minutes on ungreased pan until tops are cracked.

HEIDI'S CREAM CHEESE BARS

Ingredients

2 tubes crescent rolls	8 oz cream cheese, softened
1 egg	1 tsp vanilla
1/2 C sugar	

- Preheat oven to 350 F. Lay 1 tube of rolls in bottom of 9x11 pan.
- Mix cream cheese, egg, sugar and vanilla. (will still have some small chunks) Pour over bottom layer.
- Refrigerate until mixture is thick. Then place second tube of rolls on top.
- Bake until golden on top (10-12 minutes).
- Sprinkle powdered sugar on top.

PERFECT RICE KRISPIE BARS

Ingredients

5 T butter	6 C rice krispies
8.5 C mini marshmallows	1/2 tsp salt

- Line 9x13 pan with foil or parchment paper and spray with cooking oil.
- In large pot on low heat, melt butter. Then add 8 C marshmallows, stirring constantly.
- Once marshmallows melted, remove from heat and add cereal and salt.
- Then add last 1/2 C marshmallows and stir.
- Pour in pan and press evenly.
- Cool, cut, and enjoy!

MOLTEN LAVA CAKES

Ingredients

10 T butter	2 large egg yolks
8 oz chocolate chips, any kind	1/2 C flour
1 tsp vanilla	1.5 C powdered sugar
3 large eggs	

- Preheat oven to 425 F. Spray 6 ramekins. Melt chips and butter in microwave for 60 seconds, then 30 seconds until smooth. Stirring between.
- Add flour, sugar, eggs and yolks. Stir. Add vanilla and stir.
- Divide into ramekins and cook for 10 minutes on a baking sheet. Edges will be firm but runny in center. Sprinkle with powdered sugar on top.

FRUITY PEBBLES CHEESECAKE BITES

Ingredients

1.5 C cream cheese, softened	1/2 C fruity pebbles
1/2 C powdered sugar, optional	

- Let cream cheese come to room temp to soften.
- Place in bowl with fruity pebbles and mix well.
- Taste to see if you want extra sugar, if so add and mix to taste.
- Place into round ice cube trays.
- Freeze for at least 3 hours. Run lukewarm water on back of ice tray to pop them out.

AUNT JENNI'S MONSTER COOKIES

Ingredients

6 beaten eggs	4 tsp baking soda
2 C brown sugar	2 sticks butter, softened
2 C sugar	1.5 lbs. creamy peanut butter
1.5 tsp light corn syrup	9 C instant oatmeal
1.5 tsp vanilla	1 bag chocolate chips
	12 oz M&Ms

- In a large bowl, add each ingredient one at a time in order (down 1st column and then start at 2nd column).
- Once everything added and mixed well, cover and chill dough overnight.
- Preheat oven to 350 F. Place Tablespoon sized heaps of dough on baking sheet. Bake until tops start to brown (about 10-12 minutes) and cool on cooling racks.
  - Note: chilling the dough results in softer and better tasting cookies

1 HOUR CINNAMON ROLLS

Ingredients	
2 3/4 C flour	1/2 C water
3 T sugar	1/4 C milk
1 tsp salt	*For filling*: 1/4 C unsalted butter, softened
1 package instant yeast	2 T cinnamon
2 T unsalted butter	1/4 C brown sugar
1 large egg	

- In large bowl, mix flour, sugar, salt and yeast until evenly dispersed. Set aside.
- Heat the water, milk and butter together in microwave until butter is melted (30-45 seconds). Stir butter mix into flour mixture. Add egg and knead for 304 minutes. Place in lightly greased bowl and rest for 5 minutes.
- Preheat oven to 200 F. Turn off after 10 minutes or just before placing rolls in oven.
- After dough has rested, roll it out into a 9x15 rectangle. Spread softened butter on top. Mix cinnamon and brown sugar and sprinkle all over dough. Roll up dough tightly and cut into 9 even pieces.
- Place in lightly greased 9-inch pan and lightly cover with foil.
- Turn off the oven and place rolls in oven to rise for 20 minutes. Remove foil, leave rolls in oven and turn oven to 375 F. Bake rolls for 15-20 minutes or until golden. Remove from oven and top with icing (next recipe).

CREAM CHEESE CINNAMON ROLL ICING

Ingredients	
2 oz cream cheese	7 T butter, softened
1/2 tsp vanilla	2 T milk
1.5 C powdered sugar	1/4 tsp salt

- Beat cream cheese and butter with electric mixer in large bowl until creamy.
- Add vanilla and milk, mix well.
- Gradually add powdered sugar and salt until smooth and fluffy.
- Spread over cinnamon rolls.

Miscellaneous

- Strawberry moonshine
- Sugar body scrub
- Slush punch/Graduation punch
- Homemade ice cream
- Easy homemade spaghetti sauce
- Cinnamon sugar
- Taco seasoning
- Chili seasoning
- Italian seasoning
- Poultry seasoning
- BBQ seasoning
- Jerk seasoning

STRAWBERRY MOONSHINE

Ingredients

4 C sugar	12 C water
4 C fresh lemon juice	1.5 pints strawberry puree
5 C Everclear liquor	Mason jars

- Pour water and sugar in large pasta pot on low heat. Stir until sugar completely dissolved.
- Remove from heat and cool to room temp.
- Wash and dry strawberries. Remove stems and dice. Blend berries until smooth and pureed.
- Mix puree with lemon juice and add to sugar water.
- Add everclear and stir well.
- Strain liquor mix to remove pulp.
- Pour into mason jars and refrigerate at least 2 weeks. The longer the better.
- Can be drank straight from jar or mix with 7-up.

SUGAR BODY SCRUB

Ingredients

1/2 C coconut oil	1.5-2 C sugar
1 T desired scent (peppermint, citrus, etc.)	1 drop of desired color food coloring, optional

- Microwave coconut oil 15-25 seconds until softened.
- Start by adding 1.5 C sugar to oil with scent extract and food coloring. Mix until ingredients are well combined and coloring is evenly distributed. If mixture too wet, add another 1/2 C sugar.
- Spoon into airtight container (such as mason jar) and use daily on face/body.

SLUSH PUNCH/GRADUATION PUNCH

Ingredients

3 packets of Kool-Aid (2 in desired flavor and 1 lemon)	2 C sugar
1 1/2 C pineapple juice	2 bottles ginger ale or 7-up

- Mix all but soda in a 5-quart bucket. Fill rest of bucket with water.
- Freeze and take our 5-6 hours before serving. Add two bottles of ginger ale/7-up.
- Enjoy the slush.

HOMEMADE ICE CREAM

Ingredients

4 eggs	2 C sugar
2 cans evaporate milk	4 tsp vanilla
1/2 tsp almond flavoring	1/2 tsp salt
Gallon Vit. D milk	Ice cream maker

- Mix all but Vit. D milk and pour into ice cream maker.
- Fill with Vit. D milk until 2 inches from top.
- Pack ice machine with layers of ice and rock salt until reaches top of reservoir.
- Turn on machine, keep ice full until machine stops (45-60 minutes).
- Stir and enjoy.

EASY HOMEMADE SPAGHETTI SAUCE

Ingredients

1.5 lbs. ground beef	1 large onion, diced
1 large green pepper, chopped	2 cloves minced garlic
3 (15 oz) can diced tomatoes	1 (6 oz) can tomato paste
2 tsp brown sugar	1.5 tsp dried oregano
1 tsp salt	1/2 tsp dried basil and thyme
1 bay leaf	2 C beef broth or water

- In a dutch oven, cook meat, onion, green pepper and garlic until meat is browned and vegetables tender. Drain off fat.
- Stir in undrained tomatoes, tomato paste, brown sugar, oregano, salt, basil, thyme, and bay leaf.
- Stir in broth. Bring to a boil and reduce heat. Simmer uncovered for 1.5-2 hours or until sauce is desired consistency, stirring occasionally. Remove bay leaf.
- Serve over cooked spaghetti.

CINNAMON SUGAR	
Ingredients	
1 C sugar	1/4 to 1/3 cup cinnamon

- Mix well. Put in shaker and keep in cupboard.

TACO SEASONING	
Ingredients	
1 tsp chili powder	1/2 tsp garlic powder
1/4 tsp onion powder	1/4 tsp cayenne pepper
1/4 tsp oregano	1/2 tsp paprika
1 tsp cumin	1/2 tsp salt
1/2 tsp black pepper	

- Mix well and store in airtight container.

CHILI SEASONING	
Ingredients	
1 T chili powder	1 tsp cumin
1/4 tsp cayenne pepper	1/2 tsp garlic powder
1/2 tsp onion powder	1/4 tsp black pepper
1 tsp oregano	1/2 tsp paprika

- Mix well and store in airtight container.

ITALIAN SEASONING	
Ingredients	
1.5 tsp oregano	1 tsp parsley
1 tsp thyme	1/2 tsp basil
1/2 tsp sage	1/2 tsp salt
1/2 tsp black pepper	

- Mix well and store in airtight container.

POULTRY SEASONING

Ingredients	
2 T thyme	1 T rosemary
1 T sage	1 tsp marjoram
1/2 tsp black pepper	1/2 tsp celery seed
1/2 tsp nutmeg	

- Mix well and store in airtight container.

BBQ SEASONING

Ingredients	
1 T salt	1 T black pepper
1 T chili powder	1 T garlic powder
1 T paprika	1 T onion powder

- Mix well and store in airtight container.

JERK SEASONING

Ingredients	
2 tsp allspice	2 tsp cumin
2 tsp coconut sugar (can sub regular)	1 tsp sage
1 tsp thyme	1/2 tsp nutmeg
1/2 tsp salt	1/4 tsp cayenne pepper
Juice of 1 lime	

- Mix seasonings together and store in airtight container.
- Prior to use, juice 1 lime into seasoning, mix and rub seasoning onto meat.

Made in the USA
Columbia, SC
23 December 2019

85609508R00033